This manual provides information on the development of the ICD-10 multiaxial system and describes its structure and use. The system has three axes: Axis I – Clinical diagnoses; Axis II – Disabilities; Axis III – Contextual factors, and is intended for use in clinical, educational and research activities. It has been prepared by an international team of experts and field tested in 20 countries. The system was shown to be easy to use and applicable in a wide range of cultures and settings. The manual is accompanied by the ICD-10 Multiaxial Diagnostic Formulation Form, WHO Short Disability Assessment Schedule (WHO DAS-S) and Axis I and Axis III glossaries.

**Multiaxial Presentation of the
ICD-10 for use in Adult Psychiatry**

WORLD HEALTH ORGANIZATION

# Multiaxial Presentation of the ICD-10 for use in Adult Psychiatry

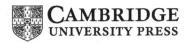
CAMBRIDGE
UNIVERSITY PRESS

CAMBRIDGE UNIVERSITY PRESS
Cambridge, New York, Melbourne, Madrid, Cape Town, Singapore, São Paulo

Cambridge University Press
The Edinburgh Building, Cambridge CB2 8RU, UK

Published in the United States of America by Cambridge University Press, New York

www.cambridge.org
Information on this title: www.cambridge.org/9780521585026

First published 1997
This digitally printed version 2007

*A catalogue record for this publication is available from the British Library*

*Library of Congress Cataloguing in Publication data*

World Health Organization.
Multiaxial presentation of the ICD-10 for use in adult psychiatry.
  p.  cm.
Edited by A. Janca and others.
Includes bibliographical references.
ISBN 0 521 58502 3 (hb)
1. Mental illness – Classification.   2. Mental illness – Diagnosis.   I. Janca, A.
[DNLM: 1. Mental Disorders – classification.   2. Mental Disorders – diagnosis.   WM 15 M961 1997]
RC455.2.C4M85   1997
616.89'001'2 – dc21   96-51767 CIP
DNLM/DLC
for Library of Congress

ISBN 978-0-521-58502-6 hardback
ISBN 978-0-521-71474-7 paperback

# Contents

# Part I

# Introduction

After more than a decade of intensive work, the Tenth Revision of the International Statistical Classification of Diseases and Related Health Problems (ICD-10) [1] has been finalized and published by the World Health Organization (WHO). It has been produced as a response to recent changes in health service systems in different parts of the world incorporating significant new knowledge that has become available in the past decade [2]. The ICD-10 consists of 21 chapters covering the whole of medical practice. Chapter V of the ICD-10 deals with mental and behavioural disorders and has been produced in several versions, each of which is intended for a particular purpose and aimed at specific users. The main versions of the *ICD-10 Classification of Mental and Behavioural Disorders* are: *Clinical Descriptions and Diagnostic Guidelines* (CDDG) [3] – an assembly of detailed specifications of the main clinical features of mental and behavioural disorders intended for general clinical, educational and service use by psychiatrists and other mental health professionals; *Diagnostic Criteria for Research* (DCR) [4] – a set of specified, operational criteria and rules intended for diagnostic purposes in research on mental and behavioural disorders; *Multiaxial Presentations of the ICD-10* – classificatory systems for the assessment of different attributes of the patient's clinical condition, designed for use in adult psychiatry and child and adolescent psychiatry [5]; *ICD-10 Primary Health Care Version* (ICD-10 PHC) [6]– a simplified list of psychiatric conditions accompanied by guidelines about diagnosis and management for use in primary health care. The ICD-10 'family' of classifications have so far been produced in equivalent versions in 36 different languages.

The recently finalized multiaxial presentation of the ICD-10 for use in adult psychiatry (hereafter ICD-10 multiaxial system) is a new member of the ICD-10 'family' of classifications and is designed as a tool for clinicians' multiaspect assessment and comprehensive formulation of the psychiatric patient's clinical condition. The ICD-10 presented as a multiaxial system uses the following axes: Axis I – Clinical diagnoses; Axis II – Disabilities; and Axis III – Contextual factors. Axis I of the outlined schema covers both the mental and physical disorders catalogued in Chapters I–XX (categories A00–Y98) of ICD-10. Axis II deals with disability due to impairments produced by the disorder(s) from which the patient suffers. It is accompanied by the WHO Short Disability Assessment Schedule (WHO DAS-S) – an instrument derived from the WHO Psychiatric Disability Assessment Schedule (WHO DAS) [7] and designed for the assessment of disabilities in the following areas of the patient's functioning: personal care; occupation; family and household; and the broader social context (e.g. leisure activities) [8]. Axis III of the system is intended for clinicians' reporting of contextual factors that influence the diagnosis, treatment or prognosis of disorders that are recorded on Axis I. It includes a selection of ICD-10 Z categories, i.e., Factors Influencing Health Status and Contact with Health Services (Chapter XXI of ICD-10) [9].

Between 1993 and 1995 the cross-cultural applicability and reliability of the ICD-10 multiaxial system were explored in two WHO-coordinated international field trials involving 274 clinicians from 20 countries spanning all the regions of the world (Africa, Asia, Europe, Latin America, North America and Oceania). About 90% of the clinicians belonging to different psychiatric schools and traditions found the ICD-10 multiaxial system to be easy to use, useful and applicable for use in their cultures and settings.

The field trials results of the ICD-10 multiaxial system indicated that there are a number of areas of its possible application across cultures and settings. The first of these areas is routine clinical work in which the ICD-10 multiaxial system could represent a useful tool for the efficient simultaneous assessment of different aspects of the patient's illness and thus better understanding of the patient's plight, impairment and surrounding circumstances. Research on mental disorders is the second area of possible application of the ICD-10 multiaxial system. The system allows more thorough, uniform and consistent collection of data and can improve the reliability and precision of the assessment and increase the consistency and comparability of the collected information. The systematic application of the ICD-10 multiaxial system could also generate a database useful in both routine clinical care and research. The extensive multiaspect coverage of the patient's illness makes the ICD-10 multiaxial system a useful teaching tool in the training of mental health professionals. The application of the system can teach a disciplined and complete review of the different aspects of the patient's illness necessary for a thorough clinical examination. Modern information processing technology makes the retrieval, organization and communication of different diagnostic statements from the ICD-10 multiaxial system easy, thus ensuring its suitability for the coding and statistical reporting of morbidity. Properly used, the multiaxial classification can also provide valuable information for epidemiological studies and for the management of health services [10].

Dr A. Janca
Dr M. Kastrup
Dr H. Katschnig
Dr J.J. López-Ibor, Jr
Dr J.E. Mezzich
Dr N. Sartorius

Dr A. Bertelsen and Dr J.E. Cooper provided the authors of this book with the most valuable comments on the presentation of the ICD-10 multiaxial system.

## References

1. World Health Organization (1992) *International Statistical Classification of Diseases and Related Health Problems, tenth revision (ICD-10)*. Geneva: World Health Organization.
2. Sartorius, N. (1995) *Understanding the ICD-10 Classification of Mental Disorders: A Pocket Reference*. London: Science Press.
3. World Health Organization (1992) *The ICD-10 Classification of Mental and Behavioural Disorders: Clinical Descriptions and Diagnostic Guidelines*. Geneva: World Health Organization.
4. World Health Organization (1993) *The ICD-10 Classification of Mental and Behavioural Disorders: Diagnostic Criteria for Research*. Geneva: World Health Organization.
5. World Health Organization (1996) *Multiaxial Classification of Child and Adolescent Psychiatric Disorders*. Cambridge: Cambridge University Press.
6. World Health Organization (1996) *Diagnostic and Management Guidelines for Mental Disorders in Primary Care: ICD-10*. Chapter V Primary Care Version. Göttingen: WHO/Hogrefe and Huber Publishers.
7. World Health Organization (1988) *WHO Psychiatric Disability Assessment Schedule (WHO/DAS)*. Geneva: World Health Organization.

8.  Janca, A., Kastrup, M., Katschnig, H., López-Ibor, J.J. Jr, Mezzich, J.E., Sartorius, N. (1996) The World Health Organization's short disability assessment schedule (WHO DAS-S): a tool for the assessment of difficulties in selected areas of functioning of patients with mental disorders. *Social Psychiatry and Psychiatric Epidemiology*, **31**, 349–54.

9.  Janca, A., Kastrup, M., Katschnig, H., López-Ibor, J.J. Jr, Mezzich, J.E., Sartorius, N. (1996) Contextual aspects of mental disorders: a proposal for axis III of the ICD-10 multiaxial system. *Acta Psychiatrica Scandinavica*, **94**, 31–6.

10. Janca, A., Kastrup, M., Katschnig, H., López-Ibor, J.J. Jr, Mezzich, J.E., Sartorius, N. (1996) The ICD-10 multiaxial system for use in adult psychiatry: structure and applications. *Journal of Nervous and Mental Disease*, **184** (3), 191–2.

# Acknowledgements

Following is a listing of the individuals and centres participating in various activities related to the development and testing of the Multiaxial Presentation of ICD-10.

Overall coordination: Dr A. Janca and Dr N. Sartorius, Geneva, Switzerland.

Members of the expert advisory committee: Dr M. Kastrup, Hvidovre, Denmark; Dr H. Katschnig, Vienna, Austria; Dr J.J. López-Ibor, Jr, Madrid, Spain; Dr J.E. Mezzich, New York (formerly Pittsburgh), USA.

Field trials data analysis: Dr L. Kirisci, Pittsburgh, USA.

Axis III definitions: Dr S. Saxena, New Delhi, India.

Directors of the field trials coordinating centres: Dr A. Bertelsen, Aarhus, Denmark; Dr D. Caetano, Campinas, Brazil; Dr S.M. Channabasavanna, Bangalore, India; Dr H. Dilling, Lübeck, Germany; Dr M. Gelder, Oxford, UK; Dr J.J. López-Ibor Jr, Madrid, Spain; Dr G. Mellsop, Wellington, New Zealand; Dr Y. Nakane, Nagasaki, Japan; Dr A. Okasha, Cairo, Egypt; Dr Ch. Pull, Luxembourg; Dr D. Regier, Rockville, USA (coordinator Dr J.E. Mezzich, Pittsburgh, USA); Dr Xu Tao-Yuan, Shanghai, China.

Field trials participants reporting to coordinating centres in:

*Aarhus, Denmark:* Dr A. Bertelsen, Aarhus; Dr R. Giel, Groningen, Netherlands; Dr A. de Jong, Groningen, Netherlands; Dr Dehelean, Timosoara, Romania; Dr O.J.K. Larsen, Frederiksberg; Dr M. Kastrup, Hvidovre.

*Bangalore, India:* Dr A.K. Agarwal, Lucknow; Dr L.N. Gupta, Udaipur; Dr S. Saxena, New Delhi; Dr R.S. Murthy, Bangalore; Dr M. Varwaese, Bangalore; Dr C. Shamasundar, Bangalore; Dr L.N. Sharma, Ranchi;

Dr V. K. Varma, Chandigarh; Dr C.R. Chandrashekar, Bangalore; Dr U. Maung Ko, Yangon, Myanmar.

*Cairo, Egypt:* Dr A. Okasha, Cairo; Dr Bahjat Abdel Rahim, Al Fhais, Jordan.

*Campinas, Brazil:* Dr M. Jorge, Sao Paulo; Dr E.D. Busnello, Porto Alegre.

*Luxembourg:* Dr J.D. Guelfi, Paris, France; Dr van Amerongen, St Germain, France; Dr Dollfus, Rouen, France.

*Lübeck, Germany:* Dr H. Biehl, Frankfurt am Main; Dr M. von Cranach, Kaufbeuren; Dr H. Dilling, Lübeck; Dr V. Dittmann, Basel, Switzerland; Dr H. Helmchen, Berlin; Dr W. Schneider, Dortmund; Dr S. Tonscheidt, Donaueschingen; Dr R.D. Stieglitz, Freiburg/Breisgau; Dr P. Hoff, München; Dr H. Katschnig, Dr M. Amering, Dr C. Klier, Dr C. Holzinger, Dr C. Müler, Dr J. Wancata, Dr J. Windhab, Dr B. Fink, Dr E. Etzesdorfer, Vienna, Austria; Dr M. Poustka, Frankfurt/Main; Dr W. Mombour, München; Dr M. Zaudig, Windach.

*Madrid, Spain:* Dr J.J. López-Ibor, Jr., Dr C. Carbonell, Dr M. Henández-Herreros, Dr A. Fernández-Liria, Dr B. Viar, Dr J. Santo-Domingo, Dr M. Delgado, Dr J.F. Durán, Dr T. Palomo, Dr C. Leal, Valencia; Dr T. Angosto, Vigo; Dr J.F. Diez-Manrique, Santander; Dr A. Medina, Córdoba; Dr J. Bobes, Oviedo; Dr S. Cervera, Pamplona; Dr F.J. Vaz, Badajoz; Dr J. Pérez de los Cobos, Barcelona; Dr M. Ruiz, Málaga; Dr J.L. González de Rivera, Tenerife; Dr J. Vallejo, Barcelona; Dr A. Rodríguez, Santiago de Compostela; Dr J.M. Mongil, Sevilla; Dr E. Peñuelas, Oviedo; Dr F. Rivas, Málaga; Dr J. Sama, Córdoba; Dr F. Lolas, Santiago de Chile; Dr A. Otero, Havana, Cuba; Dr P. Valdés, Havana, Cuba; Dr D. Warthon, Lima, Peru; Dr O. Alonso-Betancourt, Camaguey, Cuba.

*Nagasaki, Japan:* Dr Y. Nakane, Nagasaki; Dr Y. Honda, Tokyo; Dr M. Nishizono, Fukuoka; Dr Y. Okubo, Tokyo; Dr T. Takahashi, Chiba; Dr I. Yamashita, Sapporo; Dr M. Asai, Tokyo; Dr N. Yamaguchi, Kanazawa.

*Oxford, UK:* Dr M. Gelder, Oxford; Dr J. Corbett, Birmingham; Dr G.W. Fenton, Dundee; Dr J. Lucey, Beckenham; Dr V.M. Mathew, Leicester; Dr G. Milner, Worcester; Dr R. Peveler, Southampton; Dr M.A. Reveley, Leicester; Dr P. Smolik, Prague, Czech Republic; Dr P. Tyrer, London; Dr P. Wright, Beckenham.

*Rockville/Pittsburgh, USA:* Dr J.E. Mezzich, Pittsburgh, PA; Dr P. Garrido, Cambridge, MA; Dr A.F. Lehman, Baltimore, MD; Dr A. Gruenberg, Philadelphia, PA; Dr Keh-Ming Lin, Torrance, CA.

*Shanghai, China:* Dr Xu Tao-Yuan, Shanghai; Dr Shen Yu-Cun, Beijing.

*Wellington, New Zealand:* Dr G. Mellsop, Wellington; Dr E. Chiu, Melbourne, Australia; Dr P. Ellis, Wellington; Dr G. Ungvari, Rosanna, Australia; Dr P. McGorry, Melbourne, Australia.

The Axis I and Axis III glossaries in Part II of this volume are based on the World Health Organization (1992) *The Tenth Revision of the International Statistical Classification of Diseases and Related Health Problems (ICD-10)*, published by WHO, Geneva, reproduced with permission.

# Development of the ICD-10 multiaxial system

The first multiaxial system developed under WHO auspices was a multi-axial classification of mental disorders in childhood. This classification, originally produced as a companion to the ICD-8, currently uses ICD-10 diagnoses and places them in the following multiaxial framework: Axis I – Clinical psychiatric syndromes; Axis II – Specific disorders of psychological development; Axis III – Intellectual level; Axis IV– Medical conditions; Axis V – Associated abnormal psychosocial situations; and Axis VI – Global assessment of psychosocial disability.

Another multiaxial system produced and tested in the framework of a WHO study in primary care settings is a triaxial classification of problems frequently presenting in primary health care. The system was developed to facilitate and stimulate the recording of psychosocial problems in primary health care and requires that general practitioners record for each patient: (a) psychological problem(s); (b) social problem(s); (c) physical problem(s). The fact that the system was not linked to the main body of the ICD–10 made its use sporadic and less attractive.

Since a WHO meeting on the diagnosis and classification of mental disorders held in Moscow in 1969, there has been a number of recommendations regarding the development of a multiaxial classification of mental disorders in old age. The axes were to serve for the recording of the clinical psychiatric syndrome, of the type of (cognitive) impairment and of the severity of the patient's condition in general (i.e., dependence on others for survival). These proposals were not field tested because of the shortage of funds and the fact that the mental (and general) health of the elderly was until recently seen as a problem mainly concerning industrialized countries with which they can deal without involvement of WHO.

The work on the development of the ICD-10 multiaxial system for use in adult psychiatry started in the mid-1980s with the production of a preliminary draft of the schema, which was reviewed by a number of WHO experts and collaborators in different countries. Valuable suggestions were also obtained through the World Psychiatric Association (WPA) and from consultations with national psychiatric societies on ICD-10 proposals. Most of the experts suggested that the multiaxial presentation of ICD-10 should be constructed so as to be simple and easy to use in a variety of countries, cultures and settings, and by clinicians and researchers belonging to different psychiatric schools and traditions.

# Structure of the ICD-10 multiaxial system

The ICD-10 multiaxial system has the following structure: Axis I – Clinical diagnoses; Axis II – Disabilities; and Axis III – Contextual factors. Table 1 gives a schematic presentation of the ICD-10 multiaxial system including subcategories of the axes and corresponding ICD-10 codes.

Table 1. *ICD-10 multiaxial system*

| Axes | ICD-10 categories |
| --- | --- |
| I  Clinical diagnoses: | |
| Mental disorders | F00–F99 |
| Physical disorders | A00–E90 |
| | G00–Y98 |
| II  Disabilities in: | |
| Personal care | |
| Occupation | |
| Family and household | |
| Broader social context | |
| III  Contextual factors: | |
| Problems related to negative events in childhood | Z61–Z62 |
| Problems related to education and literacy | Z55 |
| Problems related to primary support group including family circumstances | Z63 |
| Problems related to the social environment | Z60 |
| Problems related to housing or economic circumstances | Z59 |
| Problems related to (un)employment | Z56 |
| Problems related to physical environment | Z57–Z58 |
| Problems related to certain psychosocial circumstances | Z64 |
| Problems related to legal circumstances | Z65 |

Table 1 (*cont.*)

| Axes | ICD-10 categories |
|---|---|
| Problems related to family history of diseases or disabilities | Z81–Z82 |
| Problems related to lifestyle and life-management difficulties | Z72–Z73 |

There are several features that distinguish the ICD-10 multiaxial system from other multiaxial classifications currently proposed: (i) according to the ICD-10 multiaxial schema, all the disorders (i.e., psychiatric, personality and physical) are to be recorded on the same axis, thus also exemplifying the principle that the distinction between mental and physical disorders is unjustified and has harmful consequences for the development of both psychiatry and medicine in general. The users are encouraged to employ as many codes as necessary to reflect the patient's clinical condition and record them as their Axis I statement; (ii) if the patient suffers from more than one disorder, the user of the ICD-10 multiaxial system is instructed to assess disability in the main areas of the patient's functioning without attempting to guess how much of it is due to each of the disorders or untoward surrounding circumstances; (iii) the choice of categories for the contextual factors that influence presentation, course or outcome of the disorder(s) has been determined by epidemiological evidence and clinical practice. The descriptions of these factors are formulated so as to be congruent with the ICD-10 Chapter XXI, which makes it possible to record them using ICD-10 Z codes.

## Axis I  Clinical diagnoses

Axis I includes clinical diagnoses of all types of disorders from which the patient suffers. It does not separate mental from 'non-mental' disorders and is based on the principle that psychiatric care is part of general medical care, and that psychiatrists, as well as other physicians, have to make a global diagnostic formulation of any patient.

Modern clinical practice has moved away from the principle of selecting only one diagnosis from a hierarchically ordered list of disorders for a single patient. The number of patients who may fulfil criteria for several disorders has been shown to be high and it is often difficult to be certain whether the patient has 'comorbid' disorders or shows several manifestations of the same disease.

ICD-10 follows the principle of diagnosis based on symptoms and their severity, frequency and clustering. It excludes, as much as possible, other (e.g., social) aspects of disorders, which may be extremely relevant for the treatment of the patient, but are not essential for the concept of the disorder or for the clinical diagnosis. In ICD-10 these other aspects of the clinical diagnosis are used in classifying disorders only when this is absolutely necessary, for example, the disability is considered as an important criterion for diagnosis of dementia, as is social isolation for diagnosis of simple schizophrenia.

ICD-10 provides an alphanumeric listing of disease categories grouped in the following chapters: Chapter I: Certain infectious and parasitic diseases (A00–B99); Chapter II: Neoplasms (C00–D48); Chapter III: Diseases of the blood and blood-forming organs and certain disorders involving the immune mechanism (D50–D89); Chapter IV: Endocrine, nutritional and metabolic diseases (E00–E90); Chapter V: Mental and behavioural disorders (F00–F99); Chapter VI: Diseases of the nervous system (G00–G99); Chapter VII: Diseases of the eye and adnexa (H00–H59); Chapter VIII: Diseases of the ear and mastoid process (H60–H95); Chapter IX: Diseases of the circulatory system (I00–I99); Chapter X: Diseases of the respiratory system (J00–J99); Chapter XI: Diseases of the digestive system (K00–K93); Chapter XII: Diseases of the skin and subcutaneous tissue (L00–L99); Chapter XIII: Diseases of the musculoskeletal system and connective tissue (M00–M99); Chapter XIV: Diseases of the genitourinary system (N00–N99); Chapter XV: Pregnancy, childbirth and the puerperium (O00–O99); Chapter XVI: Certain conditions originating in the perinatal period (P00–P96); Chapter XVII: Congenital malformations, deformations, and chromosomal abnormalities (Q00–Q99); Chapter XVIII: Symptoms, signs and abnormal clinical and laboratory findings, not elsewhere classified (R00–R99); and Chapter XIX: Injury, poisoning and certain other consequences of external causes (S00–T98). In addition to the above–listed disease categories the ICD-10 includes a list of External causes of morbidity and mortality (Chapter XX: V01–Y98) and a list of Factors influencing health status and contact with health services (Z00–Z99).

Part II of this book provides a listing and glossary definitions of ICD-10 Chapter V (F00–F99) categories of mental and behavioural disorders, as well as a list of other conditions from ICD-10 often associated with mental and behavioural disorders (i.e., selected A00–E90 and G00–Y98 categories of disease groups listed above). The clinician is encouraged to employ as many ICD-10 diagnoses and respective ICD-10 codes as necessary to reflect the patient's clinical condition and record them as the Axis I statement on the ICD-10 Multiaxial Diagnostic Formulation Form. The main diagnosis should be listed first. A coding of XX should be given where there is no clinical diagnosis in any of the listed ICD-10 categories. More detailed information regarding the use of the Axis I part of the Form is given in the respective section of the book.

## Axis II    Disabilities

This axis was conceptualized in accordance with the principles embedded in the International Classification of Impairments, Disabilities and Handicaps (ICIDH) and it serves to rate disabilities in relation to the tasks and roles expected from the individual in his/her sociocultural setting. According to ICIDH, in the context of health experience an *impairment* is any loss or abnormality of psychological, physiological or anatomical structure or function. In the context of health experience, a *disability* is any restriction or lack (resulting from an impairment) of ability to perform an activity in the manner or within the range considered normal for an individual in his/her sociocultural setting. In the context of health experience, a *handicap* is a disadvantage for a given individual, resulting from an impairment or a disability, that limits or prevents the fulfilment of a role that is normal (depending on age, sex, and social and cultural factors) for that individual.

Axis II covers the following specific areas of functioning:

### A    Personal care

Personal care should be regarded as an activity guided by social norms and conventions. It refers to personal hygiene, dressing, feeding, etc. Failure to maintain acceptable standards of personal care is likely to interfere with the patient's social participation.

In rating the disability in this area of functioning, the following should be considered:

(i)    the patient's activities concerned with the maintenance of personal hygiene and physical health (e.g., washing, shaving, keeping clothes clean, etc.);

(ii)   eating habits (e.g., regular meals, weight loss or gain, etc.);

(iii)    the patient's maintenance of personal belongings and living space.

Guiding questions are: What has the patient's personal hygiene been like? Is the patient having regular meals? How much pride does the patient take in his/her appearance? What is the patient's room like compared with the rest of the house? etc.

## B    Occupation

This area refers to expected functioning in paid activities, studying, home-making, etc. In rating the disability in this area of functioning, the following should be considered:

(i)     the patient's conformity to the work discipline;
(ii)    the quality of his/her performance at work;
(iii)   his/her motivation in maintaining the occupational role.

Guiding questions are: Does the patient go to work regularly? Does the patient like his/her job? Can the patient cope with his/her job? etc. In the case of a student or housewife, adjust the questions appropriately.

## C    Family and household

This area refers to the patient's participation in family life (e.g., marital role, parental role) and household activities (e.g., doing domestic chores, having meals together, etc.). In rating, particular attention should be given to the patient's performance in the specific sociocultural context in which he/she lives.

With regard to the patient's *marital role* the following should be considered:

(i)     the patient's communication with his/her spouse;
(ii)    the patient's ability to show affection and concern;
(iii)   the extent to which the patient is felt by the spouse to be a source of support.

In determining the severity of dysfunction, the clinician should consider if there is evidence of: any reduction in the areas of communication between the patient and the spouse; any reduction in mutual affection and support; any threat to the viability of the marriage, etc.

Guiding questions are: How would you describe your marriage? Is he/she affectionate? Can you confide in him/her? etc.

With regard to the patient's *parental role*, the following should be considered:

(i) the basic tasks and activities undertaken by the patient to ensure the health and security of the children;

(ii) the closeness of their relationship and the depth of affection for and interest shown in the children's well-being and future;

(iii) any abuse of the parental role or possibility of adverse effects on the children.

In determining the severity of the dysfunction, the clinician should consider: the patient's actual performance in childcare-related tasks; the patient's involvement in the upbringing and the lives of his/her children; and the patient's competence in approaching and relating to his/her children.

Guiding questions are: How good a parent is the patient? How close is the patient to the children? etc.

With regard to the patient's participation in *household activities*, the following should be considered:

(i) the functions and duties of the patient in maintaining the family as a viable social group;

(ii) the manner in which the patient carries out his/her roles in the family (e.g., spouse, father/mother, child).

Guiding questions: What kind of things does the patient do for the children? How does he/she take part in household activities? etc.

## D   Functioning in a broader social context

This area refers to the expected performance of the patient in relation to community members, his/her participation in leisure and other social activities, etc. The patient style of adaptation to others outside the household activities and his/her mixing with people should be considered here. The following should also be considered:

(i) the way in which the patient responds to the questions, requests and demands of people outside the household;

(ii) the patient's readiness for coexistence on an 'impersonal' level (e.g., colleagues, people in the bus or shops, etc.);

(iii) the patient's manner with people outside the household whom he/she dislikes;

(iv)  the quality and amount of contact with friends and non-household members;

(v)  the patient's engagement in leisure activities outside the household.

In determining the severity of dysfunction, the clinician should consider if there is evidence of: any lack of cooperation in social situations on the part of the patient; or any adverse consequences for the patient's social functioning, i.e., restricted social integration.

Guiding questions are: What is the patient's behaviour with strangers? How does the patient get on with people at work/school/college/with neighbours? How does the patient behave with people he/she dislikes? How much does the patient engage in extra-familial/extra-household and leisure activities? etc.

### WHO Short Disability Assessment Schedule (WHO DAS-S) and its use

Axis II is accompanied by the *Short Version of WHO Disability Assessment Schedule (WHO DAS-S)* (see Part II of the book), which has been derived from the WHO Psychiatric Disability Assessment Schedule (WHO/DAS), a semi-structured interview schedule designed for the comprehensive evaluation of the social functioning of patients with mental and in particular psychotic disorders. WHO DAS-S is a simple instrument designed for the recording of the clinician's assessment of disabilities caused by mental and physical disorders. The instrument can be administered by a clinician (e.g., psychiatrist, clinical psychologist) or other health professional (e.g., general practitioner, social worker) who has had previous experience in rating behaviour and is familiar with the use of the instrument.

The WHO DAS-S is not a questionnaire and the ratings should be based on the clinician's judgement of the information obtained from the patient; key informants such as family members; case notes or other written records; and observation of the patient. To obtain relevant information, the clinician should be familiar with the content of the specific areas of functioning covered by the instrument and, in the course of the interview, should ask appropriate questions so as to be able to assess related disabilities. In assessing the disabilities, the clinician should take into account the severity (or intensity) of the disability (e.g., the number of expected tasks and roles that have been affected) as well as its duration (i.e., the proportion of time in the past during which the disability was manifest). If a disability was severe but of brief duration, it can be rated at the same level as a less severe manifestation occupying a greater proportion of time.

Prior to the assessment of disability in the specific areas of functioning, the clinician should decide upon the period of time covered by rating. The choice will depend on the main purpose of the rating (e.g., treatment planning) or the particular situation and/or setting in which the patient has been evaluated (e.g., admission to hospital). The time period options offered by the instrument are: 'current' (i.e., at the moment of the assessment); 'last month'; 'last year' and 'other (specify)'.

The patient's disability in specific areas of functioning in the chosen time period should be evaluated against the presumed 'average' or 'normal' functioning of a person of the same sex and of comparable age and sociocultural background.

### Rating

The clinician is expected to rate disability by circling the appropriate figure on the given scale of 0 ('no disability') to 5 ('gross disability') for each of the specific areas of functioning. In case of doubt, the general rule is that the clinician should select the numerically lower step. When an individual has performed because he/she was supported by someone else (e.g., family, health worker, etc.) the actual level of disability should be rated and the box 'functioning with assistance' should be ticked.

The anchor points of the scale and their definitions are as follows:

0   No disability at any time, i.e., the patient's functioning conforms to the norms of his/her reference group or sociocultural context.
1   Deviation from the norms in the performance of one or more tasks or roles expected to be carried out by the patient in his/her sociocultural setting.
2   Deviation from the norms is conspicuous and dysfunctions interfere with social adjustment, i.e., slightly disabled most of the time or moderately disabled some of the time.
3   Deviation from the norms in most of the expected tasks and roles.
4   Deviation from the norms in all the expected tasks and roles.
5   Deviation from the norms has reached a crisis point, i.e., the patient is severely disabled all the time.

### Axis III   Contextual factors

Axis III provides an opportunity for the clinician to assess contextual factors that are considered to contribute significantly to the occurrence, presentation, course, outcome or treatment of the present mental and physical disorders recorded on Axis I or to be of clear relevance for the clinical care of the present illness episode. The contextual factors are grouped and formulated in congruence with ICD-10 Z00–Z99 categories, that is, factors influencing health status and contact with health services (Chapter XXI of ICD-10). The Z00–Z99 categories in ICD-10 are provided for occasions when circumstances other than a disease or injury classifiable to categories A00–Y89 are recorded as the reason for seeking help or when some circumstance or problem is present that influences the person's health status but is not in itself a current illness or injury.

Part II of the book provides a listing and glossary definitions of selected ICD-10 Z00–Z99 categories included as contextual factors in Axis III of the ICD-10 multiaxial system. The selection and thematic grouping of contextual factors have been based on the field trials results of the ICD-10 multiaxial system. To facilitate their use in clinical practice the categories of contextual factors in Part II have been given in the following order: problems related to negative events in childhood; problems related to education and literacy; problems related to primary support group including family circumstances; problems related to the social environment; problems related to housing or economic circumstances; problems related to (un)employment; problems related to physical environment; problems related to certain psychosocial circumstances; problems related to legal circumstances; problems related to family history of diseases or disabilities; and problems related to lifestyle and life-management difficulties.

In order to ensure common understanding of Axis III categories and to enhance reliability of their use, contextual factors have been accompanied by brief definitions that have been newly developed or modified from the definitions of specific Z codes in Chapter XXI of ICD-10.

A contextual factor should be recorded by the clinician only if it has been of such severity and duration that it has, in his/her opinion, significantly influenced the present condition of the patient or is of relevance for the clinical care of the present illness. In case of the existence of multiple contextual factors, the clinicians are encouraged to note as many of them as they judge to be relevant. The clinicians are requested to take the patient's sociocultural background into consideration when assessing the importance of a given contextual factor (e.g., death of a distant relative may be of sufficient importance to be rated positively for a patient living in the same household, but not for a patient living apart from that person in a nuclear family).

The time frame of a contextual factor also depends on clinical judgement – factors are to be recorded as present, irrespective of the time of their appearance, if judged relevant to the present illness (e.g., death of spouse several years ago should be recorded if the event is relevant to the present state; on the other hand, death of spouse a few months ago need not be recorded if the clinician did not consider it of importance for the present state of the patient). Factors of a lasting nature are also to be recorded only if they are judged important for the current condition of the patient.

Contextual factors fulfilling the criteria of an Axis I condition should not be coded on Axis III (e.g., problems regarding alcohol use). Problems considered to play merely a contributory role should not be coded on Axis III. In the case of several contextual factors, the codification of these should be listed according to their severity and influence on the present Axis I disorder.

# The ICD-10 Multiaxial Diagnostic Formulation Form and its use

The ICD-10 multiaxial assessment is a comprehensive diagnostic procedure intended to provide a biopsychosocial portrayal of the patient's clinical condition. The clinician's evaluation and the multiaxial formulation should be based on all available information about the patient, including: results of the clinical examination (both psychiatric and physical); data obtained from relatives and other informants; review of medical records, laboratory and other diagnostic tests; results of psychological testing; social worker reports; and data from other sources such as school or work reports.

The results of the clinician's multiaxial evaluation of the patient should be recorded on the ICD-10 Multiaxial Diagnostic Formulation Form, which is printed on the inside back cover. This form consists of one section for recording the basic information about the patient, clinician and assessment, and three further sections, each of which is intended for recording and rating information pertinent to specific axes of the ICD-10 multiaxial schema. Prior to the administration of the form, the clinician should decide upon the time period covered by the assessment, that is, current, last month, last year or other (specify) and indicate it on the form.

In the Axis I section of the form, the clinician should list all the positive ICD-10 diagnoses of both mental (including personality) and physical disorders and conditions. The clinician is encouraged to employ as many ICD-10 diagnoses and respective codes as reflect the patient's clinical condition. The respective ICD-10 F00–F99 categories for mental disorders and A00–E90 and G00–Y98 categories for physical disorders and conditions should be recorded under the rubric 'ICD-10 codes'. The listing of ICD-10 diagnoses and categories to be used for recording purposes is given in Part II of the book. It comprises the listing and glossary definitions of the ICD-10 categories of mental and behavioural disorders (F00–F99) and the listing of other (i.e., physical) disorders and conditions from the ICD-10 often associated with mental and behavioural disorders (selected A00–E90 and G00–Y98 categories). If the clinician cannot find the diagnosis and category in the provided list, he or she should record the clinical diagnosis and leave the rubric 'ICD-10 codes' blank. In such a case, the ICD-10 diagnosis and respective ICD-10 code should be entered later after consulting the full version of the ICD-10.

In the Axis II part of the ICD-10 Multiaxial Diagnostic Formulation Form, the clinician should transfer the ratings from the WHO DAS-S, the use of which is explained in detail with the description of Axis II of the ICD-10 multiaxial system.

The Axis III part of the ICD-10 Multiaxial Diagnostic Formulation Form is intended for recording the clinician's assessment of all the contextual factors that had played a significant role in the occurrence, presentation, course or outcome of the disorders recorded on Axis I, or that are of clear relevance for the clinical care of the patient's condition. The clinician should list all present contextual factors and enter specific Z codes for each. The factors should be listed in order of their importance. More detailed explanations regarding the assessment of severity, duration and time frame of contextual factors are given with the description of Axis III of the ICD-10 multiaxial system. A listing of contextual factors with respective Z codes and brief definitions are given in Part II of the book.

# Field trials of the ICD-10 multiaxial system

The field testing of the ICD-10 multiaxial system was organized as a WHO-coordinated project comprising two international field trials of the applicability, feasibility and reliability of the proposed ICD-10 schema. The specific objectives of the first field trial were: (i) to assess the applicability and ease of use of the ICD-10 multiaxial schema in the daily work of psychiatrists and other mental health professionals; (ii) to determine the perceived usefulness of the multiaxial presentation of ICD-10 for: (a) support of decisions regarding regular patient care; (b) training of mental health professionals; (c) research on mental disorders; and (d) statistical reporting and other public health purposes; (iii) to identify problems experienced in the use of the ICD-10 multiaxial schema; (iv) to obtain an estimate of the inter-rater reliability for each of the axes of the ICD-10 multiaxial schema. The second field trial was aimed at exploring the consequences of the amendments made to the ICD-10 multiaxial system after the analysis of results of the first field test.

The ICD-10 multiaxial field trials package consisted of the following documents: (1) Field Trials Protocol, specifying the phases of work and assessment procedures; (2) Case Study Form, intended for recording the assessment and comments of each clinician for each case; (3) Final Comments Form, intended for clinicians' overall rating of and comments on the ICD-10 multiaxial schema after their completion of the field trial; (4) ICD-10 CDDG, containing detailed descriptions of ICD-10 mental and behavioural disorders as well as a listing of other (i.e., physical) disorders and conditions that were found to be often associated with the disorders included in ICD-10 Chapter V itself; (5) WHO Disability Diagnostic Scale (WHO DDS), with brief guidelines for its use and rating instructions; (6) Listing of contextual factors and respective ICD-10 Z codes with a brief set of rules for recording their significance; and (7) 12 case vignettes containing descriptions of psychiatric patients seen in different countries.

The field trials documents were sent to 14 ICD-10 coordinating centres located in Campinas, Brazil; Shanghai, China; Aarhus, Denmark;

Cairo, Egypt; Lübeck, Germany; Bangalore, India; Naples, Italy; Nagasaki, Japan; Luxembourg, Luxembourg; Wellington, New Zealand; Moscow, Russian Federation; Madrid, Spain; Oxford, UK; and Rockville, USA. Each of these centres had undertaken to coordinate work in a number of other centres sharing the same psychiatric tradition and/or language. The coordinating centres were asked to translate and distribute these materials to the professionals and institutions who expressed interest in participating in the field trials of the ICD-10 multi-axial system.

The field work at each participating centre included the following: (1) Familiarization with the ICD-10 multiaxial schema, field trials protocol and instruments. For each participating clinician, this involved studying the pertinent materials and applying them in the assessment of five psychiatric patients. (2) Rating of 12 psychiatric case vignettes by two clinicians and completion of a Case Study Form for each case. (3) Assessment (by two clinicians making their ratings independently) of 10 general psychiatric patients selected in an unbiased way (e.g., first patient of the day) so as to yield a reasonably representative sample of the general psychiatric population cared for at each centre. (4) Formulation of final comments. At the end of the trial, participating clinicians completed the Final Comments Form indicating their views regarding the perceived usefulness of the ICD-10 multiaxial schema as a whole and formulating specific recommendations for improving it.

After completion of the field work, the participating centres sent the Case Study Forms and Final Comments Forms to the respective ICD-10 coordinating centres. These centres were provided with computerized data entry programs based on the EPI INFO computer statistical program developed by WHO. After entering the data received from the participants in their area, the coordinating centres sent diskettes to WHO in Geneva, where the data sets were assembled and cleaned. The analysis of the field trials data was completed in collaboration with the University of Pittsburgh Medical Center.

The analysis of the field trials data included a content analysis of the ratings and comments made on the Case Study Forms and Final Comments Forms and the computation of inter-rater reliability coefficients determined by using extended kappa (for agreement on Axis I and Axis III ICD-10 categories) and intraclass correlation (for Axis II disability ratings). The analyses were carried out bearing in mind (i) that the results of analyses of assessment of disabilities and pathogenetic factors in patients seen in different cultures can at best be seen as indicative;

and (ii) that the next phase of work in the development of the ICD-10 multiaxial system will be the development and testing of definitions of different levels of disabilities and of pathogenetic factors in different sociocultural settings.

### Results of Phase I of the field trials

The first field trial of the ICD-10 multiaxial system was conducted in 1993–94, with the participation of 246 clinicians from 63 centres located in 20 different countries spanning all the regions of the world (Africa, Asia, Europe, Latin America, North America and Oceania) (Table 2). A total number of 4374 assessments of local patients and case vignettes was made across the sites. The majority of the clinicians participating in the first field trial were males (81.5%) in the age group 20–40 (69.1%); 50.5% of the assessed patients were in the age group 20–40 with a slight predominance of males (57.0%) and recruits from inpatient settings (59.0%).

Table 2. *Participation in the field trials of the ICD-10 multiaxial system*

| Countries | Centres | Clinicians | Assessments |
|---|---|---|---|
| *Phase I:* | | | |
| Australia | 1 | 3 | 78 |
| Brazil | 1 | 2 | 44 |
| Chile | 1 | 2 | 24 |
| China | 2 | 6 | 88 |
| Cuba | 1 | 2 | 44 |
| Czech Republic | 1 | 8 | 176 |
| Egypt | 1 | 15 | 163 |
| France | 3 | 6 | 108 |
| Germany | 1 | 10 | 147 |
| India | 5 | 16 | 300 |
| Japan | 6 | 35 | 675 |
| Myanmar | 1 | 5 | 48 |
| Netherlands | 1 | 3 | 54 |
| New Zealand | 2 | 5 | 88 |
| Peru | 1 | 2 | 44 |
| Romania | 2 | 6 | 132 |
| Spain | 21 | 84 | 1570 |
| UK | 5 | 15 | 322 |

Table 2 (*cont.*)

| Countries | Centres | Clinicians | Assessments |
|-----------|---------|------------|-------------|
| USA | 6 | 20 | 269 |
| *Total:* | *62* | *245* | *4374* |
| *Phase II:* | | | |
| Austria | 1 | 7 | 189 |
| Denmark | 1 | 19 | 494 |
| Spain | 1 | 2 | 52 |
| *Total:* | *3* | *28* | *735* |

## Axis I   Clinical diagnoses

The frequency analysis of clinicians' ratings of Axis I categories showed that a diagnosis from the ICD-10 F2 category, i.e., Schizophrenia, schizotypal and delusional disorders, and F3 category, i.e., Mood (affective) disorders, was made in 40.1% of patients and 48.3% of case vignettes . The most frequently recorded physical disorders were from the ICD-10 G category, i.e., Diseases of the nervous system (2.1%), and Axis I category, i.e., Diseases of the circulatory system (2.1%). An average of 1.35 ICD-10 diagnoses of mental and physical disorders per patient and 1.33 per case vignette was made by the clinicians.

The overall kappa coefficient for Axis I diagnoses of mental and behavioural disorders (i.e., F categories) was 0.44 for the assessment of patients and 0.53 for the set of case vignettes, with 0.76 representing the highest kappa value obtained in the F20–F29 categories (i.e., Schizophrenia, schizotypal and delusional disorders) in the set of case vignettes. The overall kappa value for physical disorders (i.e., 'non-F' categories) recorded on Axis I was 0.59 in the patient group and 0.53 in the set of case vignettes, with the highest kappa value of 0.83 in the E00–E90 categories (i.e., Endocrine, nutritional and metabolic diseases) in the patient group and 0.85 in the V01–Y98 categories (i.e., External causes of morbidity and mortality) in the set of case vignettes. The overall kappa for all the Axis I diagnostic categories (i.e., A00–Y98 categories) was 0.58 (0.60 for the patient group and 0.57 for the case vignettes).

Axis II    Disabilities

The clinicians' ratings of Axis II categories indicated that in 69.5% of patients and 77.5% of case vignettes the 'global' disability was rated in the range of medium values of the WHO DDS, i.e., 'obvious' to 'very severe'. About half of the patients and case vignettes (43.0% and 51.4% respectively) were found to be 'very severely' or 'grossly' disabled in 'occupational functioning'; a smaller proportion of patients and cases described in the vignettes (21.7% and 33.2% respectively) were rated as 'very severely' or 'grossly' disabled in 'personal care and survival'. 'Functioning in family and household' was 'very severely' or 'grossly' affected in 33.4% of patients and 38.0% of case vignettes and disability in 'broader social context' was rated as 'very severe' or 'gross' in 39.4% of patients and 50.5% of case vignettes.

The intraclass correlation coefficients for Axis II disability categories ranged from 0.13 for disability in 'family and household activities' to 0.45 for disability in the 'broader social context' in the patient group. With the exception of intraclass correlation coefficients for disability in 'occupational activities' and 'broader social context' in the patient group (0.42 and 0.45 respectively) the intraclass correlation coefficients for all other disability categories in both the patient group and the set of case vignettes did not reach 0.40.

Axis III    Contextual factors

The most frequently rated Axis III category of contextual factors was 'problems related to primary support group including family circum-stances' (24.9% in the patient group; 27.9% in the set of case vignettes). With regard to specific contextual factors, 'problems in relationship with spouse or partner' (Z63.0) and 'problems in relationship with parents or in-laws' (Z63.1) were the most frequently rated in the patient group (5.6% and 4.4% respectively), while the 'disruption of family by separa-tion or divorce' (Z63.5) was the most frequently rated specific contextual factor in the set of case vignettes (5.8%). The average number of record-ed contextual factors per patient was 2.61 and 2.23 per case vignette.

The kappa values for the agreement between the raters on the absence and presence of significant contextual factors recorded on Axis III was 0.94 and 0.83 respectively. The kappa values for the individual Z cate-gories ranged from 0.04 for 'problems related to negative events in childhood' (Z61–Z62) to 0.57 for 'problems related to family history of diseases or disabilities' (Z81–Z82) in the patient group, and from 0.15 for 'problems related to negative events in childhood' (Z61–Z62) to 0.55 for 'problems related to education and literacy' (Z55) in the set of case vignettes. The kappa value for the most frequently recorded specific contextual factor, 'problems in relationship with spouse or partner' (Z63.0) (5.6% in the patient group, 4.3% in the set of case vignettes), was 0.64.

Ease of use and usefulness

The majority of the clinicians rated the use of the whole ICD-10 multiaxial system as being 'rather easy' (73%) or 'very easy' (17%). Similar ratings were given to the ease of use of the three axes of the schema. No significant difference in the ratings of ease of use of the ICD-10 multiaxial system existed when it was applied to assess the patients or case vignettes.

After the completion of the field trial, about 80% of the 178 clinicians (who submitted their Final Comments Forms) assigned the ICD-10 multiaxial system 'highly' or 'generally useful' for regular patient care, training of mental health professionals, research on mental disorders, statistical reporting and other public health purposes (e.g., management of health services). Only 3% of the clinicians found the system and its axes not to be useful for the above listed purposes and the remainder rated it as 'marginally useful'.

## Results of Phase II of the field trials

Taking into account the results of the first field trial as well as comments and recommendations of the field trial participants, several amendments were made to the ICD-10 multiaxial system. The forms were simplified and an improved set of instructions was produced for each of the axes of the schema. The system was accompanied by a newly developed ICD-10 Multiaxial Diagnostic Formulation Form giving a graphic presentation of the schema, rating instructions and coding columns. The WHO DDS was revised and produced as a 6-point rating scale with precise definitions of the anchor points and specifications for the assessment time frame (i.e., current; last month; last year; and other/specify). The 'functioning with assistance' box was added to each of the specific areas of functioning covered by the instrument to be able to rate the actual disabilities in patients who were able to perform some of their tasks because of the support of another person (e.g., family member, health worker). At the end of the instrument, the clinician was provided with an opportunity to rate and describe 'specific abilities' of the patient which, according to previous research and experience obtained in the first field trial, were found to be useful for the comprehensive formulation of the patient's functioning in the community. Finally, the revised instrument, which drew many of its features from the WHO DAS, was renamed as the Short Version of WHO Disability Assessment Schedule (WHO DAS-S).

A second, small-scale field trial to explore the consequences of the amendments made to the ICD-10 multiaxial system was organized in 1994–95, involving the participation of 28 clinicians and the assessment of six case vignettes and 61 patients from Austria, Denmark and Spain. With the exception of a more balanced male/female ratio of clinicians (52.4% : 47.6%), the other sociodemographic characteristics of the participants and assessed patients in the first and second phases of the field trials were not significantly different.

The analysis of data collected in the second field trial of the ICD-10 multiaxial system showed the following:

- The kappa value for all Axis I diagnoses was 0.70 in the patient group and 0.67 in the set of case vignettes; 71% of recorded F categories had kappa values of 0.50 or higher; the overall kappa value for physical disorders (i.e., 'non-F' categories) was 0.61 in the patient group and 0.54 in the set of case vignettes;
- The kappa values for the total duration of disabilities and presence of the specific abilities in the patient were 0.85 and 0.86 respectively; the intraclass correlation coefficients for specific disability categories ranged from 0.40 for disability in 'family and household activities' in the patient group to 0.74 for disability in 'personal care' in the set of case vignettes; 50% of specific disability categories had kappa values above 0.50 and for the other 50% the kappa values were in the range of 0.40 to 0.50.
- The most frequently rated specific contextual factors in this field trial were 'unemployment, unspecified' (Z56.0) and 'family history of mental disorder' (Z82.0) (5.8% and 6.4% respectively) and their kappa values in the patient group were 0.74 and 0.65 respectively; in the set of case vignettes the kappa values for these contextual factors were 0.52 and 0.62 respectively; 81% of the sizably represented specific contextual factors had kappa values of 0.70 or higher.

The content analysis of the second field trial participants' comments revealed a problem in the relationship between rating of global disability and disabilities in specific areas of functioning, that is, many clinicians could not make 'independent' assessments of the two, and rated global disability either as an average or equal to the maximum disability in the specific areas of functioning. To avoid ambiguities, most of the clinicians suggested deletion of the global disability rating.

## Comment

The ICD-10 multiaxial system for use in adult psychiatry aims to provide clinicians with a tool for the systematic assessment and a more comprehensive formulation of different aspects of the psychiatric patient's state. The schema was designed after an extensive review of the existing multiaxial systems and developed with the help of an international expert advisory committee and a large number of experts from different parts of the world, including members of the WPA, participants in the development of different versions of the ICD-10 and others collaborating in WHO programmes.

The results of the international field trials of the ICD-10 multiaxial system showed that the majority of clinicians belonging to different psychiatric schools and traditions found the schema to be user-friendly, applicable in their settings and useful in routine clinical work, training, research and statistics of mental disorders. The participants in the first field trial suggested a number of ways to improve the recording of information on specific axes of the ICD-10 multiaxial schema. The recommended amendments were incorporated in the system and tested in the second field trial, the results of which indicated that the suggested changes improved the feasibility and reliability of the schema and its axes. The second field trial also indicated the necessity for further adjustments of the schema, i.e., deletion of the Axis II 'global functioning' category and inclusion of brief glossary definitions and descriptions of the Axis I and Axis III categories, which has been done in the current version of the ICD-10 multiaxial system.

Small samples (i.e., ten patients per centre) and the uneven participation of clinicians and centres across countries (e.g., more than one-third of the participants in the first field trial were from Spanish-speaking countries; the second field trial was conducted in only three Western European countries) represent important limitations of the field testing of the ICD-10 multiaxial system. The finding of limited reliability of specific axes of the ICD-10 multiaxial system was not surprising, in view of the fact that the assessment of disabilities and contextual factors related to mental disorders requires good knowledge of the cultural setting in which the patient lives and detailed information about his or her activities and that these factors may have been explored differently across the participating centres.

Nevertheless, the field trials results demonstrated the good general acceptability of the ICD-10 multiaxial system and it seems possible to conclude that the current version of the schema represents an internationally applicable model for clinicians' multi-aspect assessment of the psychiatric patient's clinical state and of the factors relevant to its management. Bearing in mind that the Axis II and Axis III categories of the system could depend on the characteristics of local circumstances, there might be a need for modification of the system at national level (e.g., to provide culturally relevant definitions of disabilities and contextual factors).

The ICD-10 multiaxial system has now been released for general use. Although the results of the international field trials indicated its cross-cultural applicability, usefulness and improved reliability, the real test of the system will be in its routine use by clinicians in different cultures and settings. WHO will collect reports on experience with the ICD-10 multiaxial schema and its components and will take them into account in producing the next edition of the system.

The new edition of the ICD-10 multiaxial system will also benefit from the development of the operational criteria and instruments for the ICIDH, the revision of which is under way. It is expected that once further developed the ICD-10 multiaxial system could serve as a 'bridge' between the ICD-10 and ICIDH, thus enhancing the probability that the two WHO classifications will be used by clinicians and other health professionals in different parts of the world jointly and in a useful manner.

# Part II

Part II

# Axis One

## Glossary of clinical diagnoses

# One

### ICD-10 Categories of mental and behavioural disorders (F00–F99)

#### Organic, including symptomatic, mental disorders (F00–F09)

This section comprises a range of mental disorders grouped together on the basis of their having in common a demonstrable etiology in cerebral disease, brain injury, or other insult leading to cerebral dysfunction. The dysfunction may be primary, as in diseases, injuries and insults that affect the brain directly and selectively; or secondary, as in systemic diseases and disorders that attack the brain only as one of the multiple organs or systems of the body that are involved.

Dementia (F00–F03) is a syndrome due to disease of the brain, usually of a chronic or progressive nature, in which there is disturbance of multiple higher cortical functions, including memory, thinking, orientation, comprehension, calculation, learning capacity, language, and judgement. Consciousness is not clouded. The impairments of cognitive function are commonly accompanied, and occasionally preceded, by deterioration in emotional control, social behaviour, or motivation. This syndrome occurs in Alzheimer's disease, in cerebrovascular disease, and in other conditions primarily or secondarily affecting the brain.

Use additional code, if desired, to identify the underlying disease. The primary code is for the underlying disease and is marked with a dagger (†); an optional additional code for the manifestation is marked with an asterisk (*).

#### F00*   *Dementia in Alzheimer's disease (G30.–†)*
Alzheimer's disease is a primary degenerative cerebral disease of unknown etiology with characteristic neuropathological and neurochemical features. The disorder is usually insidious in onset and develops slowly but steadily over a period of several years.

#### F00.0*   *Dementia in Alzheimer's disease with early onset (G30.0 †)*
Dementia in Alzheimer's disease with onset before the age of 65, with a relatively rapid deteriorating course and with marked multiple disorders of the higher cortical functions.

- Alzheimer's disease, type 2
- Presenile dementia, Alzheimer's type

• Primary degenerative dementia of the Alzheimer's type, presenile onset

*F00.1\* Dementia in Alzheimer's disease with late onset (G30.1†)*
Dementia in Alzheimer's disease with onset after the age of 65, usually in the late 70s or thereafter, with a slow progression, and with memory impairment as the principal feature.

• Alzheimer's disease, type 1
• Primary degenerative dementia of the Alzheimer's type, senile onset
• Senile dementia, Alzheimer's type

*F00.2\* Dementia in Alzheimer's disease, atypical or mixed type (G30.8†)*
Atypical dementia, Alzheimer's type

*F00.9\* Dementia in Alzheimer's disease, unspecified (G30.9†)*

F01    *Vascular dementia*
Vascular dementia is the result of infarction of the brain due to vascular disease, including hypertensive cerebrovascular disease. The infarcts are usually small but cumulative in their effect. Onset is usually in later life.

*Includes:* • arteriosclerotic dementia

*F01.0 Vascular dementia of acute onset*
Usually develops rapidly after a succession of strokes from cerebrovascular thrombosis, embolism or haemorrhage. In rare cases, a single large infarction may be the cause.

*F01.1 Multi-infarct dementia*
Gradual in onset, following a number of transient ischaemic episodes which produce an accumulation of infarcts in the cerebral parenchyma.

• Predominantly cortical dementia

*F01.2 Subcortical vascular dementia*
Includes cases with a history of hypertension and foci of ischaemic destruction in the deep white matter of the cerebral hemispheres. The cerebral cortex is usually preserved and this contrasts with the clinical picture, which may closely resemble that of dementia in Alzheimer's disease.

*F01.3 Mixed cortical and subcortical vascular dementia*

*F01.8 Other vascular dementia*

*F01.9 Vascular dementia, unspecified*

**F02\***   *Dementia in other diseases classified elsewhere*
Cases of dementia due, or presumed to be due, to causes other than Alzheimer's disease or cerebrovascular disease. Onset may be at any time in life, though rarely in old age.

*F02.0\* Dementia in Pick's disease (G31.0†)*
A progressive dementia, commencing in middle age, characterized by early, slowly progressing changes of character and social deterioration, followed by impairment of intellect, memory, and language functions, with apathy, euphoria and, occasionally, extrapyramidal phenomena.

*F02.1\* Dementia in Creutzfeldt–Jakob disease (A81.0†)*
A progressive dementia with extensive neurological signs, due to specific neuropathological changes that are presumed to be caused by a transmissible agent. Onset is usually in middle or later life, but may be at any adult age. The course is subacute, leading to death within one to two years.

*F02.2\* Dementia in Huntington's disease (G10†)*
A dementia occurring as part of a widespread degeneration of the brain. The disorder is transmitted by a single autosomal dominant gene. Symptoms typically emerge in the third and fourth decade. Progression is slow, leading to death usually within 10 to 15 years.

* Dementia in Huntington's chorea

*F02.3\* Dementia in Parkinson's disease (G20†)*
A dementia developing in the course of established Parkinson's disease. No particular distinguishing clinical features have yet been demonstrated.

Dementia in:
* paralysis agitans
* parkinsonism

*F02.4\* Dementia in human immunodeficiency virus [HIV] disease (B22.0†)*
Dementia developing in the course of HIV disease, in the absence of a concurrent illness or condition other than HIV infection that could explain the clinical features.

*F02.8\* Dementia in other specified diseases classified elsewhere*
Dementia in:
* cerebral lipidosis (E75.–†)
* epilepsy (G40.–†)
* hepatolenticular degeneration (E83.0†)
* hypercalcaemia (E83.5†)

- hypothyroidism, acquired (E01, E03.–†)
- intoxications (T36–T65†)
- multiple sclerosis (G35†)
- neurosyphilis (A52.1†)
- niacin deficiency [pellagra] (E52†)
- polyarteritis nodosa (M30.0†)
- systemic lupus erythematosus (M32.–†)
- trypanosomiasis: (B56.–†, B57.–†)
- vitamin B12 deficiency (E53.8†)

### F03    Unspecified dementia
Presenile:
- dementia NOS
- psychosis NOS

Primary degenerative dementia NOS
Senile:
- dementia:
  - NOS
  - depressed or paranoid type
- psychosis NOS

Excludes:   • senile dementia with delirium or acute confusional state (F05.1)
            • senility NOS (R54)

### F04    Organic amnesic syndrome, not induced by alcohol and other psychoactive substances

A syndrome of prominent impairment of recent and remote memory while immediate recall is preserved, with reduced ability to learn new material and disorientation in time. Confabulation may be a marked feature, but perception and other cognitive functions, including the intellect, are usually intact. The prognosis depends on the course of the underlying lesion.

- Korsakov's psychosis or syndrome, nonalcoholic

Excludes:   amnesia:
            • NOS (R41.3)
            • anterograde (R41.1)
            • dissociative (F44.0)
            • retrograde (R41.2)
            Korsakov's syndrome:
            • alcohol-induced or unspecified (F10.6)
            • induced by other psychoactive substances
              (F11–F19 with common fourth character .6)

**F05    *Delirium, not induced by alcohol and other psychoactive substances***
An etiologically nonspecific organic cerebral syndrome characterized by concurrent disturbances of consciousness and attention, perception, thinking,
memory, psychomotor behaviour, emotion, and the sleep-wake schedule. The
duration is variable and the degree of severity ranges from mild to very severe.

*Includes:*  acute or subacute:
- brain syndrome
- confusional state (nonalcoholic)
- infective psychosis
- organic reaction
- psycho-organic syndrome

*Excludes:*  • delirium tremens, alcohol-induced or unspecified (F10.4)

**F05.0  *Delirium not superimposed on dementia, so described***

**F05.1  *Delirium superimposed on dementia***
Conditions meeting the above criteria but developing in the course of a dementia
(F00–F03)

**F05.8  *Other delirium***
Delirium of mixed origin

**F05.9  *Delirium, unspecified***

**F06    *Other mental disorders due to brain damage and dysfunction and to physical
disease***
Includes miscellaneous conditions causally related to brain disorder due to primary cerebral disease, to systemic disease affecting the brain secondarily, to
exogenous toxic substances or hormones, to endocrine disorders, or to other
somatic illnesses.

*Excludes:*  associated with:
- delirium (F05.–)
- dementia as classified in F00–F03

resulting from use of alcohol and other psychoactive substances
(F10–F19)

**F06.0  *Organic hallucinosis***
A disorder of persistent or recurrent hallucinations, usually visual or auditory,
that occur in clear consciousness and may or may not be recognized by the
subject as such. Delusional elaboration of the hallucinations may occur, but
delusions do not dominate the clinical picture; insight may be preserved.

- Organic hallucinatory state (nonalcoholic)

*Excludes:*   • alcoholic hallucinosis (F10.5)
              schizophrenia (F20.–)

### F06.1  Organic catatonic disorder

A disorder of diminished (stupor) or increased (excitement) psychomotor activity associated with catatonic symptoms. The extremes of psychomotor disturbance may alternate.

*Excludes:*   • catatonic schizophrenia (F20.2)
              • stupor:
                • NOS (R40.1)
                • dissociative (F44.2)

### F06.2  Organic delusional [schizophrenia-like] disorder

A disorder in which persistent or recurrent delusions dominate the clinical picture. The delusions may be accompanied by hallucinations. Some features suggestive of schizophrenia, such as bizarre hallucinations or thought disorder, may be present.

- Paranoid and paranoid–hallucinatory organic states
- Schizophrenia-like psychosis in epilepsy

*Excludes:*   • disorder:
              • acute and transient psychotic (F23.–)
              • persistent delusional (F22.–)
              • psychotic drug–induced (F11–F19 with common fourth character .5)
              • schizophrenia (F20.–)

### F06.3  Organic mood [affective] disorders

Disorders characterized by a change in mood or affect, usually accompanied by a change in the overall level of activity, depressive, hypomanic, manic or bipolar (see F30–F32), but arising as a consequence of an organic disorder.

*Excludes:*   • mood disorders, nonorganic or unspecified (F30–F39)

### F06.4  Organic anxiety disorder

A disorder characterized by the essential descriptive features of a generalized anxiety disorder (F41.1), a panic disorder (F41.0), or a combination of both, but arising as a consequence of an organic disorder.

*Excludes:*   • anxiety disorders, nonorganic or unspecified (F41.–)

### F06.5  Organic dissociative disorder

A disorder characterized by a partial or complete loss of the normal integration between memories of the past, awareness of identity and immediate sensations, and control of bodily movements (see F44.–), but arising as a consequence of an organic disorder.

*Excludes:* • dissociative [conversion] disorders, nonorganic or
             un-specified (F44.–)

### F06.6  Organic emotionally labile [asthenic] disorder

A disorder characterized by emotional incontinence or lability, fatigability, and a variety of unpleasant physical sensations (e.g. dizziness) and pains, but arising as a consequence of an organic disorder.

*Excludes:* • somatoform disorders, nonorganic or unspecified (F45.–)

### F06.7  Mild cognitive disorder

A disorder characterized by impairment of memory, learning difficulties, and reduced ability to concentrate on a task for more than brief periods. There is often a marked feeling of mental fatigue when mental tasks are attempted, and new learning is found to be subjectively difficult even when objectively success-ful. None of these symptoms is so severe that a diagnosis of either dementia (F00–F03) or delirium (F05.–) can be made. This diagnosis should be made only in association with a specified physical disorder, and should not be made in the presence of any of the mental or behavioural disorders classified to F10–F99. The disorder may precede, accompany, or follow a wide variety of infections and physical disorders, both cerebral and systemic, but direct evidence of cerebral involvement is not necessarily present. It can be differentiated from posten-cephalitic syndrome (F07.1) and postconcussional syndrome (F07.2) by its dif-ferent etiology, more restricted range of generally milder symptoms, and usually shorter duration.

### F06.8  Other specified mental disorders due to brain damage and dysfunction and to physical disease

Epileptic psychosis NOS

### F06.9  Unspecified mental disorder due to brain damage and dysfunction and to physical disease

Organic:
• brain syndrome NOS
• mental disorder NOS

## F07  Personality and behavioural disorders due to brain disease, damage and dysfunction

Alteration of personality and behaviour can be a residual or concomitant disor-der of brain disease, damage or dysfunction.

*F07.0  Organic personality disorder*
A disorder characterized by a significant alteration of the habitual patterns of behaviour displayed by the subject premorbidly, involving the expression of emotions, needs and impulses. Impairment of cognitive and thought functions, and altered sexuality may also be part of the clinical picture.

Organic:
• pseudopsychopathic personality
• pseudoretarded personality
Syndrome:
• frontal lobe
• limbic epilepsy personality
• lobotomy
• postleucotomy
*Excludes:*  • enduring personality change after:
         • catastrophic experience (F62.0)
         • psychiatric illness (F62.1)
       • postconcussional syndrome (F07.2)
       • postencephalitic syndrome (F07.1)
       • specific personality disorder (F60.–)

*F07.1  Postencephalitic syndrome*
Residual nonspecific and variable behavioural change following recovery from either viral or bacterial encephalitis. The principal difference between this disorder and the organic personality disorders is that it is reversible.

*Excludes:*  • organic personality disorder (F07.0)

*F07.2  Postconcussional syndrome*
A syndrome that occurs following head trauma (usually sufficiently severe to result in loss of consciousness) and includes a number of disparate symptoms such as headache, dizziness, fatigue, irritability, difficulty in concentration and performing mental tasks, impairment of memory, insomnia, and reduced tolerance to stress, emotional excitement, or alcohol.

• Postcontusional syndrome (encephalopathy)
• Post-traumatic brain syndrome, nonpsychotic

*F07.8  Other organic personality and behavioural disorders due to brain disease, damage and dysfunction*
• Right hemispheric organic affective disorder

*F07.9  Unspecified organic personality and behavioural disorder due to brain disease, damage and dysfunction*
• Organic psychosyndrome

*F09 Unspecified organic or symptomatic mental disorder*
Psychosis:

* organic NOS
* symptomatic NOS

*Excludes:* • psychosis NOS (F29)

## Mental and behavioural disorders due to psychoactive substance use (F10–F19)

This section contains a wide variety of disorders that differ in severity and clinical form but that are all attributable to the use of one or more psychoactive substances, which may or may not have been medically prescribed. The third character of the code identifies the substance involved, and the fourth character specifies the clinical state. The codes should be used, as required, for each substance specified, but it should be noted that not all fourth-character codes are applicable to all substances.

Identification of the psychoactive substance should be based on as many sources of information as possible. These include self-report data, analysis of blood and other body fluids, characteristic physical and psychological symptoms, clinical signs and behaviour, and other evidence such as a drug being in the patient's possession or reports from informed third parties. Many drug users take more than one type of psychoactive substance. The main diagnosis should be classified, whenever possible, according to the substance or class of substances that has caused or contributed most to the presenting clinical syndrome. Other diagnoses should be coded when other psychoactive substances have been taken in intoxicating amounts (common fourth character .0) or to the extent of causing harm (common fourth character .1), dependence (common fourth character .2) or other disorders (common fourth character .3–.9).

Only in cases in which patterns of psychoactive substance-taking are chaotic and indiscriminate, or in which the contributions of different psychoactive substances are inextricably mixed, should the diagnosis of disorders resulting from multiple drug use (F19.–) be used.

*Excludes:* • abuse of non-dependence-producing substances (F55)

The following fourth-character subdivisions are for use with categories F10–F19:

*.0 Acute intoxication*
A condition that follows the administration of a psychoactive substance resulting in disturbances in level of consciousness, cognition, perception, affect or behaviour, or other psycho-physiological functions and responses. The disturbances are directly related to the acute pharmacological effects of the substance and resolve with time, with complete recovery, except where tissue damage or other

complications have arisen. Complications may include trauma, inhalation of vomitus, delirium, coma, convulsions, and other medical complications. The nature of these complications depends on the pharmacological class of substance and mode of administration.

- Acute drunkenness in alcoholism
- 'Bad trips' (drugs)
- Drunkenness NOS
- Pathological intoxication
- Trance and possession disorders in psychoactive substance intoxication

### .1 Harmful use
A pattern of psychoactive substance use that is causing damage to health. The damage may be physical (as in cases of hepatitis from the self-administration of injected psychoactive substances) or mental (e.g. episodes of depressive disorder secondary to heavy consumption of alcohol).

- Psychoactive substance abuse

### .2 Dependence syndrome
A cluster of behavioural, cognitive, and physiological phenomena that develop after repeated substance use and that typically include a strong desire to take the drug, difficulties in controlling its use, persisting in its use despite harmful consequences, a higher priority given to drug use than to other activities and obligations, increased tolerance, and sometimes a physical withdrawal state.

The dependence syndrome may be present for a specific psychoactive substance (e.g. tobacco, alcohol, or diazepam), for a class of substances (e.g. opioid drugs), or for a wider range of pharmacologically different psychoactive substances.

- Chronic alcoholism
- Dipsomania
- Drug addiction

### .3 Withdrawal state
A group of symptoms of variable clustering and severity occurring on absolute or relative withdrawal of a psychoactive substance after persistent use of that substance. The onset and course of the withdrawal state are time-limited and are related to the type of psychoactive substance and dose being used immediately before cessation or reduction of use. The withdrawal state may be complicated by convulsions.

### .4 Withdrawal state with delirium
A condition where the withdrawal state as defined in the common fourth character .3 is complicated by delirium as defined in F05.–. Convulsions may also

occur. When organic factors are also considered to play a role in the etiology, the condition should be classified to F05.8.

- Delirium tremens (alcohol–induced)

### .5 Psychotic disorder

A cluster of psychotic phenomena that occur during or following psychoactive substance use but that are not explained on the basis of acute intoxication alone and do not form part of a withdrawal state. The disorder is characterized by hallucinations (typically auditory, but often in more than one sensory modality), perceptual distortions, delusions (often of a paranoid or persecutory nature), psychomotor disturbances (excitement or stupor), and an abnormal affect, which may range from intense fear to ecstasy. The sensorium is usually clear but some degree of clouding of consciousness, though not severe confusion, may be present.

Alcoholic:
- hallucinosis
- jealousy
- paranoia
- psychosis NOS

Excludes: • alcohol- or other psychoactive substance-induced residual and late-onset psychotic disorder (F10–F19 with common fourth character .7)

### .6 Amnesic syndrome

A syndrome associated with chronic prominent impairment of recent and remote memory. Immediate recall is usually preserved and recent memory is characteristically more disturbed than remote memory. Disturbances of time sense and ordering of events are usually evident, as are difficulties in learning new material. Confabulation may be marked but is not invariably present. Other cognitive functions are usually relatively well preserved and amnesic defects are out of proportion to other disturbances.

- Amnestic disorder, alcohol- or drug-induced
- Korsakov's psychosis or syndrome, alcohol- or other psychoactive substance-induced or unspecified

Excludes: • nonalcoholic Korsakov's psychosis or syndrome (F04)

### .7 Residual and late-onset psychotic disorder

A disorder in which alcohol- or psychoactive substance-induced changes of cognition, affect, personality, or behaviour persist beyond the period during which a direct psychoactive substance-related effect might reasonably be assumed to be operating. Onset of the disorder should be directly related to the use of the psychoactive substance. Cases in which initial onset of the state occurs later than episode(s) of such substance use should be coded here only where clear and strong evidence is available to attribute the state to the residual effect of the psychoactive substance. Flashbacks may be distinguished from psychotic state partly by their episodic nature, frequently of very short duration, and by their duplication of previous alcohol- or other psychoactive substance-related experiences.

- Alcoholic dementia NOS
- Chronic alcoholic brain syndrome
- Dementia and other milder forms of persisting impairment of cognitive functions
- Flashbacks
- Late-onset psychoactive substance-induced psychotic disorder
- Posthallucinogen perception disorder

Residual:

- affective disorder
- disorder of personality and behaviour

*Excludes:*  •  alcohol- or psychoactive substance-induced:
- Korsakov's syndrome (F10–F19 with common fourth character .6)
- psychotic state (F10–F19 with common fourth character .5)

*.8  Other mental and behavioural disorders*

*.9  Unspecified mental and behavioural disorder*

**F10.–**    *Mental and behavioural disorders due to use of alcohol*

**F11.–**    *Mental and behavioural disorders due to use of opioids*

**F12.–**    *Mental and behavioural disorders due to use of cannabinoids*

**F13.–**    *Mental and behavioural disorders due to use of sedatives or hypnotics*

**F14.–**    *Mental and behavioural disorders due to use of cocaine*

**F15.–**    *Mental and behavioural disorders due to use of other stimulants, including caffeine*

**F16.–**    *Mental and behavioural disorders due to use of hallucinogens*

**F17.–**    *Mental and behavioural disorders due to use of tobacco*

**F18.–**    *Mental and behavioural disorders due to use of volatile solvents*

*F19.–*   *Mental and behavioural disorders due to multiple drug use and use of other*
         *psychoactive substances*
         This category should be used when two or more psychoactive substances are
         known to be involved, but it is impossible to assess which substance is contribut-
         ing most to the disorders. It should also be used when the exact identity of some
         or even all the psychoactive substances being used is uncertain or unknown,
         since many multiple drug users themselves often do not know the details of what
         they are taking.

         *Includes:*   • misuse of drugs NOS


         **Schizophrenia, schizotypal and delusional disorders**
         **(F20–F29)**

         This section brings together schizophrenia, as the most important member of the
         group, schizotypal disorder, persistent delusional disorders, and a larger group of
         acute and transient psychotic disorders. Schizoaffective disorders have been
         retained here in spite of their controversial nature.


*F20*   *Schizophrenia*
         The schizophrenic disorders are characterized in general by fundamental and
         characteristic distortions of thinking and perception, and affects that are inappro-
         priate or blunted. Clear consciousness and intellectual capacity are usually main-
         tained although certain cognitive deficits may evolve in the course of time. The
         most important psychopathological phenomena include thought echo; thought
         insertion or withdrawal; thought broadcasting; delusional perception and delu-
         sions of control; influence or passivity; hallucinatory voices commenting or dis-
         cussing the patient in the third person; thought disorders and negative symptoms.
            The course of schizophrenic disorders can be either continuous, or episodic
         with progressive or stable deficit, or there can be one or more episodes with
         complete or incomplete remission. The diagnosis of schizophrenia should not be
         made in the presence of extensive depressive or manic symptoms unless it is
         clear that schizophrenic symptoms antedate the affective disturbance. Nor
         should schizophrenia be diagnosed in the presence of overt brain disease or dur-
         ing states of drug intoxication or withdrawal. Similar disorders developing in the
         presence of epilepsy or other brain disease should be classified under F06.2, and
         those induced by psychoactive substances under F10–F19 with common fourth
         character .5.

         *Excludes:*   schizophrenia:
                      • acute (undifferentiated) (F23.2)
                      • cyclic (F25.2)
                      schizophrenic reaction (F23.2)
                      schizotypal disorder (F21)

### F20.0  Paranoid schizophrenia
Paranoid schizophrenia is dominated by relatively stable, often paranoid delusions, usually accompanied by hallucinations, particularly of the auditory variety, and perceptual disturbances. Disturbances of affect, volition and speech, and catatonic symptoms, are either absent or relatively inconspicuous.

Paraphrenic schizophrenia
*Excludes:*   • involutional paranoid state (F22.8)
              • paranoia (F22.0)

### F20.1  Hebephrenic schizophrenia
A form of schizophrenia in which affective changes are prominent, delusions and hallucinations fleeting and fragmentary, behaviour irresponsible and unpredictable, and mannerisms common. The mood is shallow and inappropriate, thought is disorganized, and speech is incoherent. There is a tendency to social isolation. Usually the prognosis is poor because of the rapid development of 'negative' symptoms, particularly flattening of affect and loss of volition. Hebephrenia should normally be diagnosed only in adolescents or young adults.

• Disorganized schizophrenia
• Hebephrenia

### F20.2  Catatonic schizophrenia
Catatonic schizophrenia is dominated by prominent psychomotor disturbances that may alternate between extremes such as hyperkinesis and stupor, or automatic obedience and negativism. Constrained attitudes and postures may be maintained for long periods. Episodes of violent excitement may be a striking feature of the condition. The catatonic phenomena may be combined with a dream-like (oneiroid) state with vivid scenic hallucinations.
Catatonic stupor

Schizophrenic:
• catalepsy
• catatonia
• flexibilitas cerea

### F20.3  Undifferentiated schizophrenia
Psychotic conditions meeting the general diagnostic criteria for schizophrenia but not conforming to any of the subtypes in F20.0–F20.2, or exhibiting the features of more than one of them without a clear predominance of a particular set of diagnostic characteristics.

Atypical schizophrenia
*Excludes:*   • acute schizophrenia-like psychotic disorder (F23.2)
              • chronic undifferentiated schizophrenia (F20.5)
              • post-schizophrenic depression (F20.4)

*F20.4  Post-schizophrenic depression*

A depressive episode, which may be prolonged, arising in the aftermath of a schizophrenic illness. Some schizophrenic symptoms, either 'positive' or 'negative', must still be present but they no longer dominate the clinical picture. These depressive states are associated with an increased risk of suicide. If the patient no longer has any schizophrenic symptoms, a depressive episode should be diagnosed (F32.–). If schizophrenic symptoms are still florid and prominent, the diagnosis should remain that of the appropriate schizophrenic subtype (F20.0–F20.3).

*F20.5  Residual schizophrenia*

A chronic stage in the development of a schizophrenic illness in which there has been a clear progression from an early stage to a later stage characterized by long-term, though not necessarily irreversible, 'negative' symptoms, e.g. psychomotor slowing; underactivity; blunting of affect; passivity and lack of initiative; poverty of quantity or content of speech; poor nonverbal communication by facial expression, eye contact, voice modulation and posture; poor self-care and social performance.

- Chronic undifferentiated schizophrenia
- Restzustand (schizophrenic)
- Schizophrenic residual state

*F20.6  Simple schizophrenia*

A disorder in which there is an insidious but progressive development of oddities of conduct, inability to meet the demands of society, and decline in total performance. The characteristic negative features of residual schizophrenia (e.g. blunting of affect and loss of volition) develop without being preceded by any overt psychotic symptoms.

*F20.8  Other schizophrenia*

Cenesthopathic schizophrenia
Schizophreniform:
- disorder NOS
- psychosis NOS
*Excludes:* • brief schizophreniform disorders (F23.2)

*F20.9  Schizophrenia, unspecified*

**F21  Schizotypal disorder**

A disorder characterized by eccentric behaviour and anomalies of thinking and affect which resemble those seen in schizophrenia, though no definite and characteristic schizophrenic anomalies occur at any stage. The symptoms may include a cold or inappropriate affect; anhedonia; odd or eccentric behaviour; a tendency to social withdrawal; paranoid or bizarre ideas not amounting to true delusions; obsessive ruminations; thought disorder and perceptual disturbances; occasional transient quasi-psychotic episodes with intense illusions, auditory or other hallucinations, and delusion-like ideas, usually occurring without external provocation. There is no definite onset and evolution and course are usually those of a personality disorder.

Latent schizophrenic reaction
Schizophrenia:
• borderline
• latent
• prepsychotic
• prodromal
• pseudoneurotic
• pseudopsychopathic
Schizotypal personality disorder
*Excludes:* • Asperger's syndrome (F84.5)
          • schizoid personality disorder (F60.1)


### F22    *Persistent delusional disorders*

Includes a variety of disorders in which long-standing delusions constitute the only, or the most conspicuous, clinical characteristic and which cannot be classified as organic, schizophrenic or affective. Delusional disorders that have lasted for less than a few months should be classified, at least temporarily, under F23.–.

#### F22.0  *Delusional disorder*

A disorder characterized by the development either of a single delusion or of a set of related delusions that are usually persistent and sometimes lifelong. The content of the delusion or delusions is very variable. Clear and persistent auditory hallucinations (voices), schizophrenic symptoms such as delusions of control and marked blunting of affect, and definite evidence of brain disease are all incompatible with this diagnosis. However, the presence of occasional or transitory auditory hallucinations, particularly in elderly patients, does not rule out this diagnosis, provided that they are not typically schizophrenic and form only a small part of the overall clinical picture.

Paranoia
Paranoid:
• psychosis
• state
Paraphrenia (late)
Sensitiver Beziehungswahn
*Excludes:* • paranoid:
          • personality disorder (F60.0)

- psychosis, psychogenic (F23.3)
- reaction (F23.3)
- schizophrenia (F20.0)

*F22.8  Other persistent delusional disorders*

Disorders in which the delusion or delusions are accompanied by persistent hallucinatory voices or by schizophrenic symptoms that do not justify a diagnosis of schizophrenia (F20.–).

- Delusional dysmorphophobia
- Involutional paranoid state
- Paranoia querulans

*F22.9  Persistent delusional disorder, unspecified*

**F23  Acute and transient psychotic disorders**

A heterogeneous group of disorders characterized by the acute onset of psychotic symptoms such as delusions, hallucinations, and perceptual disturbances, and by the severe disruption of ordinary behaviour. Acute onset is defined as a crescendo development of a clearly abnormal clinical picture in about two weeks or less. For these disorders there is no evidence of organic causation. Perplexity and puzzlement are often present but disorientation for time, place and person is not persistent or severe enough to justify a diagnosis of organically caused delirium (F05.–). Complete recovery usually occurs within a few months, often within a few weeks or even days. If the disorder persists, a change in classification will be necessary. The disorder may or may not be associated with acute stress, defined as usually stressful events preceding the onset by one to two weeks.

*F23.0  Acute polymorphic psychotic disorder without symptoms of schizophrenia*

An acute psychotic disorder in which hallucinations, delusions or perceptual disturbances are obvious but markedly variable, changing from day to day or even from hour to hour. Emotional turmoil with intense transient feelings of happiness or ecstasy, or anxiety and irritability, is also frequently present. The polymorphism and instability are characteristic for the overall clinical picture and the psychotic features do not justify a diagnosis of schizophrenia (F20.–). These disorders often have an abrupt onset, developing rapidly within a few days, and they frequently show a rapid resolution of symptoms with no recurrence. If the symptoms persist the diagnosis should be changed to persistent delusional disorder (F22.–).

- Bouffée délirante without symptoms of schizophrenia or unspecified
- Cycloid psychosis without symptoms of schizophrenia or unspecified

*F23.1  Acute polymorphic psychotic disorder with symptoms of schizophrenia*

An acute psychotic disorder in which the polymorphic and unstable clinical picture is present, as described in F23.0; despite this instability, however, some symptoms typical of schizophrenia are also in evidence for the majority of the time. If the schizophrenic symptoms persist the diagnosis should be changed to schizophrenia (F20.–).

- Bouffée délirante with symptoms of schizophrenia
- Cycloid psychosis with symptoms of schizophrenia

### F23.2 Acute schizophrenia-like psychotic disorder

An acute psychotic disorder in which the psychotic symptoms are comparatively stable and justify a diagnosis of schizophrenia, but have lasted for less than about one month; the polymorphic unstable features, as described in F23.0, are absent. If the schizophrenic symptoms persist the diagnosis should be changed to schizophrenia (F20.–).

Acute (undifferentiated) schizophrenia
Brief schizophreniform:
- disorder
- psychosis
Oneirophrenia
Schizophrenic reaction
*Excludes:*  • organic delusional [schizophrenia-like] disorder (F06.2)
  • schizophreniform disorders NOS (F20.8)

### F23.3  Other acute predominantly delusional psychotic disorders

Acute psychotic disorders in which comparatively stable delusions or hallucinations are the main clinical features, but do not justify a diagnosis of schizophrenia (F20.–). If the delusions persist the diagnosis should be changed to persistent delusional disorder (F22.–).

- Paranoid reaction
- Psychogenic paranoid psychosis

### F23.8  Other acute and transient psychotic disorders

Any other specified acute psychotic disorders for which there is no evidence of organic causation and which do not justify classification to F23.0–F23.3.

### F23.9  Acute and transient psychotic disorder, unspecified

- Brief reactive psychosis NOS
- Reactive psychosis

## F24    Induced delusional disorder

A delusional disorder shared by two or more people with close emotional links. Only one of the people suffers from a genuine psychotic disorder; the delusions are induced in the other(s) and usually disappear when the people are separated.

Folie à deux
Induced:
• paranoid disorder
• psychotic disorder

*F25*    ***Schizoaffective disorders***
Episodic disorders in which both affective and schizophrenic symptoms are prominent but which do not justify a diagnosis of either schizophrenia or depressive or manic episodes. Other conditions in which affective symptoms are superimposed on a pre-existing schizophrenic illness, or co-exist or alternate with persistent delusional disorders of other kinds, are classified under F20–F29. Mood-incongruent psychotic symptoms in affective disorders do not justify a diagnosis of schizoaffective disorder.

*F25.0  Schizoaffective disorder, manic type*
A disorder in which both schizophrenic and manic symptoms are prominent so that the episode of illness does not justify a diagnosis of either schizophrenia or a manic episode. This category should be used for both a single episode and a recurrent disorder in which the majority of episodes are schizoaffective, manic type.

• Schizoaffective psychosis, manic type
• Schizophreniform psychosis, manic type

*F25.1  Schizoaffective disorder, depressive type*
A disorder in which both schizophrenic and depressive symptoms are prominent so that the episode of illness does not justify a diagnosis of either schizophrenia or a depressive episode. This category should be used for both a single episode and a recurrent disorder in which the majority of episodes are schizoaffective, depressive type.

• Schizoaffective psychosis, depressive type
• Schizophreniform psychosis, depressive type

*F25.2  Schizoaffective disorder, mixed type*
• Cyclic schizophrenia
• Mixed schizophrenic and affective psychosis

*F25.8  Other schizoaffective disorders*

*F25.9  Schizoaffective disorder, unspecified*
• Schizoaffective psychosis NOS

*F28*    *Other nonorganic psychotic disorders*
Delusional or hallucinatory disorders that do not justify a diagnosis of schizophrenia (F20.–), persistent delusional disorders (F22.–), acute and transient psychotic disorders (F23.–), psychotic types of manic episode (F30.2), or severe depressive episode (F32.3).

   • Chronic hallucinatory psychosis

*F29*    *Unspecified nonorganic psychosis*
Psychosis NOS
*Excludes:*  • mental disorder NOS (F99)
             • organic or symptomatic psychosis NOS (F09)

**Mood [affective] disorders**
**(F30–F39)**

This section contains disorders in which the fundamental disturbance is a change in affect or mood to depression (with or without associated anxiety) or to elation. The mood change is usually accompanied by a change in the overall level of activity; most of the other symptoms are either secondary to, or easily understood in the context of, the change in mood and activity. Most of these disorders tend to be recurrent and the onset of individual episodes can often be related to stressful events or situations.

*F30*    *Manic episode*
All the subdivisions of this category should be used only for a single episode. Hypomanic or manic episodes in individuals who have had one or more previous affective episodes (depressive, hypomanic, manic, or mixed) should be coded as bipolar affective disorder (F31.–).

*Includes:* bipolar disorder, single manic episode

*F30.0 Hypomania*
A disorder characterized by a persistent mild elevation of mood, increased energy and activity, and usually marked feelings of well-being and both physical and mental efficiency. Increased sociability, talkativeness, over-familiarity, increased sexual energy, and a decreased need for sleep are often present but not to the extent that they lead to severe disruption of work or result in social rejection. Irritability, conceit, and boorish behaviour may take the place of the more usual euphoric sociability. The disturbances of mood and behaviour are not accompanied by hallucinations or delusions.

*F30.1 Mania without psychotic symptoms*
Mood is elevated out of keeping with the patient's circumstances and may vary from carefree joviality to almost uncontrollable excitement. Elation is accompanied by increased energy, resulting in overactivity, pressure of speech, and a

decreased need for sleep. Attention cannot be sustained, and there is often marked distractibility. Self-esteem is often inflated with grandiose ideas and overconfidence. Loss of normal social inhibitions may result in behaviour that is reckless, foolhardy, or inappropriate to the circumstances, and out of character.

### F30.2 Mania with psychotic symptoms
In addition to the clinical picture described in F30.1, delusions (usually grandiose) or hallucinations (usually of voices speaking directly to the patient) are present, or the excitement, excessive motor activity, and flight of ideas are so extreme that the subject is incomprehensible or inaccessible to ordinary communication.

Mania with:
• mood-congruent psychotic symptoms
• mood-incongruent psychotic symptoms
Manic stupor

### F30.8 Other manic episodes

### F30.9 Manic episode, unspecified
• Mania NOS

## F31  Bipolar affective disorder
A disorder characterized by two or more episodes in which the patient's mood and activity levels are significantly disturbed, this disturbance consisting on some occasions of an elevation of mood and increased energy and activity (hypomania or mania) and on others of a lowering of mood and decreased energy and activity (depression). Repeated episodes of hypomania or mania only are classified as bipolar (F31.8).

Includes:  • manic-depressive:
           • illness
           • psychosis
           • reaction
Excludes:  • bipolar disorder, single manic episode (F30.–)
           • cyclothymia (F34.0)

### F31.0  Bipolar affective disorder, current episode hypomanic
The patient is currently hypomanic, and has had at least one other affective episode (hypomanic, manic, depressive, or mixed) in the past.

### F31.1  Bipolar affective disorder, current episode manic without psychotic symptoms
The patient is currently manic, without psychotic symptoms (as in F30.1), and has had at least one other affective episode (hypomanic, manic, depressive, or mixed) in the past.

*F31.2  Bipolar affective disorder, current episode manic with psychotic symptoms*
The patient is currently manic, with psychotic symptoms (as in F30.2), and has had at least one other affective episode (hypomanic, manic, depressive, or mixed) in the past.

*F31.3  Bipolar affective disorder, current episode mild or moderate depression*
The patient is currently depressed, as in a depressive episode of either mild or moderate severity (F32.0 or F32.1), and has had at least one authenticated hypomanic, manic, or mixed affective episode in the past.

*F31.4  Bipolar affective disorder, current episode severe depression without psychotic symptoms*
The patient is currently depressed, as in severe depressive episode without psychotic symptoms (F32.2), and has had at least one authenticated hypomanic, manic, or mixed affective episode in the past.

*F31.5  Bipolar affective disorder, current episode severe depression with psychotic symptoms*
The patient is currently depressed, as in severe depressive episode with psychotic symptoms (F32.3), and has had at least one authenticated hypomanic, manic, or mixed affective episode in the past.

*F31.6  Bipolar affective disorder, current episode mixed*
The patient has had at least one authenticated hypomanic, manic, depressive, or mixed affective episode in the past, and currently exhibits either a mixture or a rapid alteration of manic and depressive symptoms.

*Excludes:*  • single mixed affective episode (F38.0)

*F31.7  Bipolar affective disorder, currently in remission*
The patient has had at least one authenticated hypomanic, manic, or mixed affective episode in the past, and at least one other affective episode (hypomanic, manic, depressive, or mixed) in addition, but is not currently suffering from any significant mood disturbance, and has not done so for several months. Periods of remission during prophylactic treatment should be coded here.

*F31.8  Other bipolar affective disorders*
• Bipolar II disorder
• Recurrent manic episodes

*F31.9  Bipolar affective disorder, unspecified*

**F32  *Depressive episode***
In typical mild, moderate, or severe depressive episodes, the patient suffers from lowering of mood, reduction of energy, and decrease in activity. Capacity for

enjoyment, interest, and concentration is reduced, and marked tiredness after even minimum effort is common. Sleep is usually disturbed and appetite diminished. Self-esteem and self-confidence are almost always reduced and, even in the mild form, some ideas of guilt or worthlessness are often present. The lowered mood varies little from day to day, is unresponsive to circumstances and may be accompanied by so-called 'somatic' symptoms, such as loss of interest and pleasurable feelings, waking in the morning several hours before the usual time, depression worst in the morning, marked psychomotor retardation, agitation, loss of appetite, weight loss, and loss of libido. Depending upon the number and severity of the symptoms, a depressive episode may be specified as mild, moderate or severe.

*Includes:*    single episodes of:
- depressive reaction
- psychogenic depression
- reactive depression

*Excludes:*   • adjustment disorder (F43.2)
- recurrent depressive disorder (F33.–)
- when associated with conduct disorders in F91.– (F92.0)

### F32.0 Mild depressive episode
Two or three of the above symptoms are usually present. The patient is usually distressed by these but will probably be able to continue with most activities.

### F32.1 Moderate depressive episode
Four or more of the above symptoms are usually present and the patient is likely to have great difficulty in continuing with ordinary activities.

### F32.2 Severe depressive episode without psychotic symptoms
An episode of depression in which several of the above symptoms are marked and distressing, typically loss of self-esteem and ideas of worthlessness or guilt. Suicidal thoughts and acts are common and a number of 'somatic' symptoms are usually present.

- Agitated depression
- Major depression      } single episode without psychotic symptoms
- Vital depression

### F32.3 Severe depressive episode with psychotic symptoms
An episode of depression as described in F32.2, but with the presence of hallucinations, delusions, psychomotor retardation, or stupor so severe that ordinary social activities are impossible; there may be danger to life from suicide, dehydration, or starvation. The hallucinations and delusions may or may not be mood-congruent.

Single episodes of:
- major depression with psychotic symptoms
- psychogenic depressive psychosis
- psychotic depression
- reactive depressive psychosis

### F32.8 Other depressive episodes
- Atypical depression
- Single episodes of 'masked' depression NOS

### F32.9 Depressive episode, unspecified
- Depression NOS
- Depressive disorder NOS

## F33  Recurrent depressive disorder

A disorder characterized by repeated episodes of depression as described for depressive episode (F32.–), without any history of independent episodes of mood elevation and increased energy (mania). There may, however, be brief episodes of mild mood elevation and overactivity (hypomania) immediately after a depressive episode, sometimes precipitated by antidepressant treatment. The more severe forms of recurrent depressive disorder (F33.2 and F33.3) have much in common with earlier concepts such as manic-depressive depression, melancholia, vital depression and endogenous depression. The first episode may occur at any age from childhood to old age, the onset may be either acute or insidious, and the duration varies from a few weeks to many months. The risk that a patient with recurrent depressive disorder will have an episode of mania never disappears completely, however many depressive episodes have been experienced. If such an episode does occur, the diagnosis should be changed to bipolar affective disorder (F31.–).

Includes:  recurrent episodes of:
- depressive reaction
- psychogenic depression
- reactive depression
seasonal depressive disorder
Excludes:  • recurrent brief depressive episodes (F38.1)

### F33.0 Recurrent depressive disorder, current episode mild
A disorder characterized by repeated episodes of depression, the current episode being mild, as in F32.0, and without any history of mania.

### F33.1 Recurrent depressive disorder, current episode moderate
A disorder characterized by repeated episodes of depression, the current episode being of moderate severity, as in F32.1, and without any history of mania.

### F33.2 Recurrent depressive disorder, current episode severe without psychotic symptoms

A disorder characterized by repeated episodes of depression, the current episode being severe without psychotic symptoms, as in F32.2, and without any history of mania.

- Endogenous depression without psychotic symptoms
- Major depression, recurrent without psychotic symptoms
- Manic-depressive psychosis, depressed type without psychotic symptoms
- Vital depression, recurrent without psychotic symptoms

### F33.3 Recurrent depressive disorder, current episode severe with psychotic symptoms

A disorder characterized by repeated episodes of depression, the current episode being severe with psychotic symptoms, as in F32.3, and with no previous episodes of mania.

Endogenous depression with psychotic symptoms
Manic-depressive psychosis, depressed type with psychotic symptoms
Recurrent severe episodes of:
- major depression with psychotic symptoms
- psychogenic depressive psychosis
- psychotic depression
- reactive depressive psychosis

### F33.4 Recurrent depressive disorder, currently in remission

The patient has had two or more depressive episodes as described in F33.0–F33.3, in the past, but has been free from depressive symptoms for several months.

### F33.8 Other recurrent depressive disorders

### F33.9 Recurrent depressive disorder, unspecified

Monopolar depression NOS

## F34 Persistent mood [affective] disorders

Persistent and usually fluctuating disorders of mood in which the majority of the individual episodes are not sufficiently severe to warrant being described as hypomanic or mild depressive episodes. Because they last for many years, and sometimes for the greater part of the patient's adult life, they involve considerable distress and disability. In some instances, recurrent or single manic or depressive episodes may become superimposed on a persistent affective disorder.

### F34.0 Cyclothymia

A persistent instability of mood involving numerous periods of depression and mild elation, none of which is sufficiently severe or prolonged to justify a diagnosis of bipolar affective disorder (F31.–) or recurrent depressive disorder (F33.–). This disorder is frequently found in the relatives of patients with bipolar affective disorder. Some patients with cyclothymia eventually develop bipolar affective disorder.

• Affective personality disorder
• Cycloid personality
• Cyclothymic personality

### F34.1 Dysthymia
A chronic depression of mood, lasting at least several years, which is not sufficiently severe, or in which individual episodes are not sufficiently prolonged, to justify a diagnosis of severe, moderate, or mild recurrent depressive disorder (F33.–).

Depressive:
• neurosis
• personality disorder
Neurotic depression
Persistent anxiety depression
*Excludes:* • anxiety depression (mild or not persistent) (F41.2)

### F34.8 Other persistent mood [affective] disorders

### F34.9 Persistent mood [affective] disorder, unspecified

### F38     Other mood [affective] disorders
Any other mood disorders that do not justify classification to F30–F34, because they are not of sufficient severity or duration.

### F38.0  Other single mood [affective] disorders
• Mixed affective episode

### F38.1  Other recurrent mood [affective] disorders
• Recurrent brief depressive episodes

### F38.8  Other specified mood [affective] disorders

### F39     Unspecified mood [affective] disorder
• Affective psychosis NOS

### Neurotic, stress-related and somatoform disorders

### (F40–F48)

*Excludes:* • when associated with conduct disorder in F91.– (F92.8)

### F40    *Phobic anxiety disorders*

A group of disorders in which anxiety is evoked only, or predominantly, in certain well-defined situations that are not currently dangerous. As a result these situations are characteristically avoided or endured with dread. The patient's concern may be focused on individual symptoms like palpitations or feeling faint and is often associated with secondary fears of dying, losing control, or going mad. Contemplating entry to the phobic situation usually generates anticipatory anxiety. Phobic anxiety and depression often coexist. Whether two diagnoses, phobic anxiety and depressive episode, are needed, or only one, is determined by the time course of the two conditions and by therapeutic considerations at the time of consultation.

#### F40.0  *Agoraphobia*

A fairly well-defined cluster of phobias embracing fears of leaving home, entering shops, crowds and public places, or travelling alone in trains, buses or planes. Panic disorder is a frequent feature of both present and past episodes. Depressive and obsessional symptoms and social phobias are also commonly present as subsidiary features. Avoidance of the phobic situation is often prominent, and some agoraphobics experience little anxiety because they are able to avoid their phobic situations.

- Agoraphobia without history of panic disorder
- Panic disorder with agoraphobia

#### F40.1  *Social phobias*

Fear of scrutiny by other people leading to avoidance of social situations. More pervasive social phobias are usually associated with low self-esteem and fear of criticism. They may present as a complaint of blushing, hand tremor, nausea, or urgency of micturition, the patient sometimes being convinced that one of these secondary manifestations of their anxiety is the primary problem. Symptoms may progress to panic attacks.

- Anthropophobia
- Social neurosis

#### F40.2  *Specific (isolated) phobias*

Phobias restricted to highly specific situations such as proximity to particular animals, heights, thunder, darkness, flying, closed spaces, urinating or defecating in public toilets, eating certain foods, dentistry, or the sight of blood or injury. Though the triggering situation is discrete, contact with it can evoke panic as in agoraphobia or social phobia.

- Acrophobia
- Animal phobias
- Claustrophobia
- Simple phobia

*Excludes:* • dysmorphophobia (nondelusional) (F45.2)
            • nosophobia (F45.2)

### F40.8 Other phobic anxiety disorders

### F40.9 Phobic anxiety disorder, unspecified
• Phobia NOS
• Phobic state NOS

**F41    Other anxiety disorders**
Disorders in which manifestation of anxiety is the major symptom and is not restricted to any particular environmental situation. Depressive and obsessional symptoms, and even some elements of phobic anxiety, may also be present, provided that they are clearly secondary or less severe.

### F41.0  Panic disorder [episodic paroxysmal anxiety]
The essential feature is recurrent attacks of severe anxiety (panic), which are not restricted to any particular situation or set of circumstances and are therefore unpredictable. As with other anxiety disorders, the dominant symptoms include sudden onset of palpitations, chest pain, choking sensations, dizziness, and feelings of unreality (depersonalization or derealization). There is often also a secondary fear of dying, losing control, or going mad. Panic disorder should not be given as the main diagnosis if the patient has a depressive disorder at the time the attacks start; in these circumstances the panic attacks are probably secondary to depression.

Panic:
• attack
• state
*Excludes:* • panic disorder with agoraphobia (F40.0)

### F41.1  Generalized anxiety disorder
Anxiety that is generalized and persistent but not restricted to, or even strongly predominating in, any particular environmental circumstances (i.e. it is 'free-floating'). The dominant symptoms are variable but include complaints of persistent nervousness, trembling, muscular tensions, sweating, lightheadedness, palpitations, dizziness, and epigastric discomfort. Fears that the patient or a relative will shortly become ill or have an accident are often expressed.

Anxiety:
• neurosis
• reaction
• state
*Excludes:* • neurasthenia (F48.0)

### F41.2  Mixed anxiety and depressive disorder
This category should be used when symptoms of anxiety and depression are both present, but neither is clearly predominant, and neither type of symptom is present to the extent that justifies a diagnosis if considered separately. When both anxiety and depressive symptoms are present and severe enough to justify individual diagnoses, both diagnoses should be recorded and this category should not be used.

• Anxiety depression (mild or not persistent)

### F41.3  Other mixed anxiety disorders
Symptoms of anxiety mixed with features of other disorders in F42–F48. Neither type of symptom is severe enough to justify a diagnosis if considered separately.

### F41.8  Other specified anxiety disorders
• Anxiety hysteria

### F41.9  Anxiety disorder, unspecified
• Anxiety NOS

## F42    Obsessive-compulsive disorder
The essential feature is recurrent obsessional thoughts or compulsive acts. Obsessional thoughts are ideas, images, or impulses that enter the patient's mind again and again in a stereotyped form. They are almost invariably distressing and the patient often tries, unsuccessfully, to resist them. They are, however, recognized as his or her own thoughts, even though they are involuntary and often repugnant. Compulsive acts or rituals are stereotyped behaviours that are repeated again and again. They are not inherently enjoyable, nor do they result in the completion of inherently useful tasks. Their function is to prevent some objectively unlikely event, often involving harm to or caused by the patient, which he or she fears might otherwise occur. Usually, this behaviour is recognized by the patient as pointless or ineffectual and repeated attempts are made to resist. Anxiety is almost invariably present. If compulsive acts are resisted the anxiety gets worse.

Includes:    • anankastic neurosis
             • obsessive-compulsive neurosis
Excludes:    • obsessive-compulsive personality (disorder) (F60.5)

### F42.0  Predominantly obsessional thoughts or ruminations
These may take the form of ideas, mental images, or impulses to act, which are nearly always distressing to the subject. Sometimes the ideas are an indecisive,

endless consideration of alternatives, associated with an inability to make trivial but necessary decisions in day-to-day living. The relationship between obsessional ruminations and depression is particularly close and a diagnosis of obsessive-compulsive disorder should be preferred only if ruminations arise or persist in the absence of a depressive episode.

*F42.1 Predominantly compulsive acts [obsessional rituals]*
The majority of compulsive acts are concerned with cleaning (particularly handwashing), repeated checking to ensure that a potentially dangerous situation has not been allowed to develop, or orderliness and tidiness. Underlying the overt behaviour is a fear, usually of danger either to or caused by the patient, and the ritual is an ineffectual or symbolic attempt to avert that danger.

*F42.2 Mixed obsessional thoughts and acts*

*F42.8 Other obsessive-compulsive disorders*

*F42.9 Obsessive-compulsive disorder, unspecified*

*F43*    *Reaction to severe stress, and adjustment disorders*
This category differs from others in that it includes disorders identifiable on the basis of not only symptoms and course but also the existence of one or other of two causative influences: an exceptionally stressful life event producing an acute stress reaction, or a significant life change leading to continued unpleasant circumstances that result in an adjustment disorder. Although less severe psychosocial stress ('life events') may precipitate the onset or contribute to the presentation of a very wide range of disorders classified elsewhere in this chapter, its etiological importance is not always clear and in each case will be found to depend on individual, often idiosyncratic, vulnerability, i.e. the life events are neither necessary nor sufficient to explain the occurrence and form of the disorder. In contrast, the disorders brought together here are thought to arise always as a direct consequence of acute severe stress or continued trauma. The stressful events or the continuing unpleasant circumstances are the primary and overriding causal factor and the disorder would not have occurred without their impact. The disorders in this section can thus be regarded as maladaptive responses to severe or continued stress, in that they interfere with successful coping mechanisms and therefore lead to problems of social functioning.

*F43.0 Acute stress reaction*
A transient disorder that develops in an individual without any other apparent mental disorder in response to exceptional physical and mental stress and that usually subsides within hours or days. Individual vulnerability and coping capacity play a role in the occurrence and severity of acute stress reactions. The symptoms show a typically mixed and changing picture and include an initial

state of 'daze' with some constriction of the field of consciousness and narrow-ing of attention, inability to comprehend stimuli, and disorientation. This state may be followed either by further withdrawal from the surrounding situation (to the extent of a dissociative stupor – F44.2), or by agitation and over-activity (flight reaction or fugue). Autonomic signs of panic anxiety (tachycardia, sweat-ing, flushing) are commonly present. The symptoms usually appear within min-utes of the impact of the stressful stimulus or event, and disappear within two to three days (often within hours). Partial or complete amnesia (F44.0) for the episode may be present. If the symptoms persist, a change in diagnosis should be considered.

Acute:
- crisis reaction
- reaction to stress
Combat fatigue
Crisis state
Psychic shock

### F43.1 Post-traumatic stress disorder
Arises as a delayed or protracted response to a stressful event or situation (of either brief or long duration) of an exceptionally threatening or catastrophic nature, which is likely to cause pervasive distress in almost anyone. Predisposing factors, such as personality traits (e.g. compulsive, asthenic) or previous history of neurotic illness, may lower the threshold for the development of the syndrome or aggravate its course, but they are neither necessary nor sufficient to explain its occurrence. Typical features include episodes of repeated reliving of the trauma in intrusive memories ('flashbacks'), dreams or nightmares, occurring against the persisting background of a sense of 'numbness' and emotional blunting, detachment from other people, unresponsiveness to surroundings, anhedonia, and avoidance of activities and situations reminiscent of the trauma. There is usually a state of autonomic hyperarousal with hypervigilance, an enhanced star-tle reaction, and insomnia. Anxiety and depression are commonly associated with the above symptoms and signs, and suicidal ideation is not infrequent. The onset follows the trauma with a latency period that may range from a few weeks to months. The course is fluctuating but recovery can be expected in the majority of cases. In a small proportion of cases the condition may follow a chronic course over many years, with eventual transition to an enduring personality change (F62.0).

- Traumatic neurosis

### F43.2 Adjustment disorders
States of subjective distress and emotional disturbance, usually interfering with social functioning and performance, arising in the period of adaptation to a significant life change or a stressful life event. The stressor may have affected

the integrity of an individual's social network (bereavement, separation experiences) or the wider system of social supports and values (migration, refugee status), or represented a major developmental transition or crisis (going to school, becoming a parent, failure to attain a cherished personal goal, retirement). Individual predisposition or vulnerability plays an important role in the risk of occurrence and the shaping of the manifestations of adjustment disorders, but it is nevertheless assumed that the condition would not have arisen without the stressor. The manifestations vary and include depressed mood, anxiety or worry (or mixture of these), a feeling of inability to cope, plan ahead, or continue in the present situation, as well as some degree of disability in the performance of daily routine. Conduct disorders may be an associated feature, particularly in adolescents. The predominant feature may be a brief or prolonged depressive reaction, or a disturbance of other emotions and conduct.

- Culture shock
- Grief reaction
- Hospitalism in children

*Excludes:* • separation anxiety disorder of childhood (F93.0)

**F43.8  *Other reactions to severe stress***

**F43.9  *Reaction to severe stress, unspecified***

**F44   *Dissociative [conversion] disorders***
The common themes that are shared by dissociative or conversion disorders are a partial or complete loss of the normal integration between memories of the past, awareness of identity and immediate sensations, and control of bodily movements. All types of dissociative disorders tend to remit after a few weeks or months, particularly if their onset is associated with a traumatic life event. More chronic disorders, particularly paralyses and anaesthesias, may develop if the onset is associated with insoluble problems or interpersonal difficulties. These disorders have previously been classified as various types of 'conversion hysteria'. They are presumed to be psychogenic in origin, being associated closely in time with traumatic events, insoluble and intolerable problems, or disturbed relationships. The symptoms often represent the patient's concept of how a physical illness would be manifest. Medical examination and investigation do not reveal the presence of any known physical or neurological disorder. In addition, there is evidence that the loss of function is an expression of emotional conflicts or needs. The symptoms may develop in close relationship to psychological stress, and often appear suddenly. Only disorders of physical functions normally under voluntary control and loss of sensations are included here. Disorders involving pain and other complex physical sensations mediated by the autonomic nervous system are classified under somatization disorder (F45.0). The possibility of the later appearance of serious physical or psychiatric disorders should always be kept in mind.

*Includes:* • conversion:
            • hysteria
            • reaction
            hysteria
            hysterical psychosis
*Excludes:* • malingering [conscious simulation] (Z76.5)

### F44.0 Dissociative amnesia

The main feature is loss of memory, usually of important recent events, that is not due to organic mental disorder, and is too great to be explained by ordinary forgetfulness or fatigue. The amnesia is usually centred on traumatic events, such as accidents or unexpected bereavements, and is usually partial and selective. Complete and generalized amnesia is rare, and is usually part of a fugue (F44.1). If this is the case, the disorder should be classified as such. The diagnosis should not be made in the presence of organic brain disorders, intoxication, or excessive fatigue.

*Excludes:* • alcohol- or other psychoactive substance-induced amnesic
             disorder (F10–F19 with common fourth character .6)
         • amnesia:
         • NOS (R41.3)
         • anterograde (R41.1)
         • retrograde (R41.2)
         • nonalcoholic organic amnesic syndrome (F04)
         • postictal amnesia in epilepsy (G40.–)

### F44.1 Dissociative fugue

Dissociative fugue has all the features of dissociative amnesia, plus purposeful travel beyond the usual everyday range. Although there is amnesia for the period of the fugue, the patient's behaviour during this time may appear completely normal to independent observers.

*Excludes:* • postictal fugue in epilepsy (G40.–)

### F44.2 Dissociative stupor

Dissociative stupor is diagnosed on the basis of a profound diminution or absence of voluntary movement and normal responsiveness to external stimuli such as light, noise, and touch, but examination and investigation reveal no evidence of a physical cause. In addition, there is positive evidence of psychogenic causation in the form of recent stressful events or problems.

*Excludes:* • organic catatonic disorder (F06.1)
            stupor:
         • NOS (R40.1)
         • catatonic (F20.2)

- depressive (F31–F33)
- manic (F30.2)

### F44.3 Trance and possession disorders
Disorders in which there is a temporary loss of the sense of personal identity and full awareness of the surroundings. Include here only trance states that are involuntary or unwanted, occurring outside religious or culturally accepted situations.

*Excludes:*   states associated with:
- acute and transient psychotic disorders (F23.–)
- organic personality disorder (F07.0)
- postconcussional syndrome (F07.2)
- psychoactive substance intoxication (F10–F19 with common fourth character .0)
- schizophrenia (F20.–)

### F44.4 Dissociative motor disorders
In the commonest varieties there is loss of ability to move the whole or a part of a limb or limbs. There may be close resemblance to almost any variety of ataxia, apraxia, akinesia, aphonia, dysarthria, dyskinesia, seizures, or paralysis.

Psychogenic:
- aphonia
- dysphonia

### F44.5 Dissociative convulsions
Dissociative convulsions may mimic epileptic seizures very closely in terms of movements, but tongue-biting, bruising due to falling, and incontinence of urine are rare, and consciousness is maintained or replaced by a state of stupor or trance.

### F44.6 Dissociative anaesthesia and sensory loss
Anaesthetic areas of skin often have boundaries that make it clear that they are associated with the patient's ideas about bodily functions, rather than medical knowledge. There may be differential loss between the sensory modalities which cannot be due to a neurological lesion. Sensory loss may be accompanied by complaints of paraesthesia. Loss of vision and hearing are rarely total in dissociative disorders.

- Psychogenic deafness

### F44.7 Mixed dissociative [conversion] disorders
Combination of disorders specified in F44.0–F44.6

### F44.8 Other dissociative [conversion] disorders
Ganser's syndrome
Multiple personality
Psychogenic:

- confusion
- twilight state

*F44.9  Dissociative [conversion] disorder, unspecified*

**F45  Somatoform disorders**

The main feature is repeated presentation of physical symptoms together with persistent requests for medical investigations, in spite of repeated negative findings and reassurances by doctors that the symptoms have no physical basis. If any physical disorders are present, they do not explain the nature and extent of the symptoms or the distress and preoccupation of the patient.

*Excludes:* • dissociative disorders (F44.–)
- hair-plucking (F98.4)
- lalling (F80.0)
- lisping (F80.8)
- nail-biting (F98.8)
- psychological or behavioural factors associated with disorders or diseases classified elsewhere (F54)
- sexual dysfunction, not caused by organic disorder or disease (F52.–)
- thumb-sucking (F98.8)
- tic disorders (in childhood and adolescence) (F95.–)
- Tourette's syndrome (F95.2)
- trichotillomania (F63.3)

*F45.0  Somatization disorder*

The main features are multiple, recurrent and frequently changing physical symptoms of at least two years' duration. Most patients have a long and complicated history of contact with both primary and specialist medical care services, during which many negative investigations or fruitless exploratory operations may have been carried out. Symptoms may be referred to any part or system of the body. The course of the disorder is chronic and fluctuating, and is often associated with disruption of social, interpersonal, and family behaviour. Short-lived (less than two years) and less striking symptom patterns should be classified under undifferentiated somatoform disorder (F45.1).

Multiple psychosomatic disorder
*Excludes:* • malingering [conscious simulation] (Z76.5)

*F45.1  Undifferentiated somatoform disorder*

When somatoform complaints are multiple, varying and persistent, but the complete and typical clinical picture of somatization disorder is not fulfilled, the diagnosis of undifferentiated somatoform disorder should be considered.

- Undifferentiated psychosomatic disorder

### F45.2  Hypochondriacal disorder

The essential feature is a persistent preoccupation with the possibility of having one or more serious and progressive physical disorders. Patients manifest persistent somatic complaints or a persistent preoccupation with their physical appearance. Normal or commonplace sensations and appearances are often interpreted by patients as abnormal and distressing, and attention is usually focused upon only one or two organs or systems of the body. Marked depression and anxiety are often present, and may justify additional diagnoses.

- Body dysmorphic disorder
- Dysmorphophobia (nondelusional)
- Hypochondriacal neurosis
- Hypochondriasis
- Nosophobia

*Excludes:*  • delusional dysmorphophobia (F22.8)
            • fixed delusions about bodily functions or shape (F22.–)

### F45.3 Somatoform autonomic dysfunction

Symptoms are presented by the patient as if they were due to a physical disorder of a system or organ that is largely or completely under autonomic innervation and control, i.e. the cardiovascular, gastrointestinal, respiratory and urogenital systems. The symptoms are usually of two types, neither of which indicates a physical disorder of the organ or system concerned. First, there are complaints based upon objective signs of autonomic arousal, such as palpitations, sweating, flushing, tremor, and expression of fear and distress about the possibility of a physical disorder. Second, there are subjective complaints of a nonspecific or changing nature such as fleeting aches and pains, sensations of burning, heaviness, tightness, and feelings of being bloated or distended, which are referred by the patient to a specific organ or system.

Cardiac neurosis
Da Costa's syndrome
Gastric neurosis
Neurocirculatory asthenia
Psychogenic forms of:
- aerophagy
- cough
- diarrhoea
- dyspepsia
- dysuria
- flatulence
- hiccough
- hyperventilation
- increased frequency of micturition

- irritable bowel syndrome
- pylorospasm

*Excludes:* • psychological and behavioural factors associated with disorders or
diseases classified elsewhere (F54)

### F45.4 Persistent somatoform pain disorder

The predominant complaint is of persistent, severe, and distressing pain, which
cannot be explained fully by a physiological process or a physical disorder, and
which occurs in association with emotional conflict or psychosocial problems
that are sufficient to allow the conclusion that they are the main causative influences. The result is usually a marked increase in support and attention, either
personal or medical. Pain presumed to be of psychogenic origin occurring during the course of depressive disorders or schizophrenia should not be included
here.

Psychalgia
Psychogenic:
- backache
- headache

Somatoform pain disorder

*Excludes:* • backache NOS (M54.9)
        pain:
- NOS (R52.9)
- acute (R52.0)
- chronic (R52.2)
- intractable (R52.1)
        tension headache (G44.2)

### F45.8 Other somatoform disorders

Any other disorders of sensation, function and behaviour, not due to physical
disorders, which are not mediated through the autonomic nervous system, which
are limited to specific systems or parts of the body, and which are closely associated in time with stressful events or problems.

Psychogenic:
- dysmenorrhoea
- dysphagia, including "globus hystericus"
- pruritus
- torticollis

Teeth-grinding

### F45.9 Somatoform disorder, unspecified

Psychosomatic disorder NOS

## F48    *Other neurotic disorders*

### F48.0 Neurasthenia

Considerable cultural variations occur in the presentation of this disorder, and two main types occur, with substantial overlap. In one type, the main feature is a complaint of increased fatigue after mental effort, often associated with some decrease in occupational performance or coping efficiency in daily tasks. The mental fatiguability is typically described as an unpleasant intrusion of distracting associations or recollections, difficulty in concentrating, and generally inefficient thinking. In the other type, the emphasis is on feelings of bodily or physical weakness and exhaustion after only minimal effort, accompanied by a feeling of muscular aches and pains and inability to relax. In both types a variety of other unpleasant physical feelings is common, such as dizziness, tension headaches, and feelings of general instability. Worry about decreasing mental and bodily well-being, irritability, anhedonia, and varying minor degrees of both depression and anxiety are all common. Sleep is often disturbed in its initial and middle phases but hypersomnia may also be prominent.

- Fatigue syndrome

Use additional code, if desired, to identify previous physical illness.

*Excludes:*  • asthenia NOS (R53)
- burn-out (Z73.0)
- malaise and fatigue (R53)
- postviral fatigue syndrome (G93.3)
- psychasthenia (F48.8)

### F48.1 Depersonalization–derealization syndrome

A rare disorder in which the patient complains spontaneously that his or her mental activity, body, and surroundings are changed in their quality, so as to be unreal, remote, or automatized. Among the varied phenomena of the syndrome, patients complain most frequently of loss of emotions and feelings of estrangement or detachment from their thinking, their body, or the real world. In spite of the dramatic nature of the experience, the patient is aware of the unreality of the change. The sensorium is normal and the capacity for emotional expression intact. Depersonalization–derealization symptoms may occur as part of a diagnosable schizophrenic, depressive, phobic, or obsessive-compulsive disorder. In such cases the diagnosis should be that of the main disorder.

### F48.8 Other specified neurotic disorders

- Briquet's disorder
- Dhat syndrome
- Occupational neurosis, including writer's cramp

Psychasthenia
Psychasthenic neurosis
Psychogenic syncope

**F48.9  Neurotic disorder, unspecified**
Neurosis NOS

**Behavioural syndromes associated with physiological disturbances and physical factors (F50–F59)**

F50     **Eating disorders**
        *Excludes:*  • anorexia NOS (R63.0)
                        feeding:
                        • difficulties and mismanagement (R63.3)
                        • disorder of infancy or childhood (F98.2)
                        polyphagia (R63.2)

**F50.0  Anorexia nervosa**
A disorder characterized by deliberate weight loss, induced and sustained by the patient. It occurs most commonly in adolescent girls and young women, but adolescent boys and young men may also be affected, as may children approaching puberty and older women up to the menopause. The disorder is associated with a specific psychopathology whereby a dread of fatness and flabbiness of body contour persists as an intrusive overvalued idea, and the patients impose a low weight threshold on themselves. There is usually undernutrition of varying severity with secondary endocrine and metabolic changes and disturbances of bodily function. The symptoms include restricted dietary choice, excessive exercise, induced vomiting and purgation, and use of appetite suppressants and diuretics.

*Excludes:*  • loss of appetite (R63.0)
                • psychogenic (F50.8)

**F50.1  Atypical anorexia nervosa**
Disorders that fulfil some of the features of anorexia nervosa but in which the overall clinical picture does not justify that diagnosis. For instance, one of the key symptoms, such as amenorrhoea or marked dread of being fat, may be absent in the presence of marked weight loss and weight-reducing behaviour. This diagnosis should not be made in the presence of known physical disorders associated with weight loss.

### F50.2 Bulimia nervosa

A syndrome characterized by repeated bouts of overeating and an excessive preoccupation with the control of body weight, leading to a pattern of overeating followed by vomiting or use of purgatives. This disorder shares many psychological features with anorexia nervosa, including an overconcern with body shape and weight. Repeated vomiting is likely to give rise to disturbances of body electrolytes and physical complications. There is often, but not always, a history of an earlier episode of anorexia nervosa, the interval ranging from a few months to several years.

Bulimia NOS
Hyperorexia nervosa

### F50.3 Atypical bulimia nervosa

Disorders that fulfil some of the features of bulimia nervosa, but in which the overall clinical picture does not justify that diagnosis. For instance, there may be recurrent bouts of overeating and overuse of purgatives without significant weight change, or the typical overconcern about body shape and weight may be absent.

### F50.4 Overeating associated with other psychological disturbances

Overeating due to stressful events, such as bereavement, accident, childbirth, etc.

Psychogenic overeating
*Excludes:* • obesity (E66.–)

### F50.5 Vomiting associated with other psychological disturbances

Repeated vomiting that occurs in dissociative disorders (F44.–) and hypochondriacal disorder (F45.2), and that is not solely due to conditions classified outside this chapter. This subcategory may also be used in addition to O21.– (excessive vomiting in pregnancy) when emotional factors are predominant in the causation of recurrent nausea and vomiting in pregnancy.

Psychogenic vomiting
*Excludes:* • nausea (R11)
                • vomiting NOS (R11)

### F50.8 Other eating disorders

Pica in adults
Psychogenic loss of appetite
*Excludes:* • pica of infancy and childhood (F98.3)

### F50.9 Eating disorder, unspecified

**F51     *Nonorganic sleep disorders***
In many cases, a disturbance of sleep is one of the symptoms of another disorder, either mental or physical. Whether a sleep disorder in a given patient is an independent condition or simply one of the features of another disorder classified elsewhere, either in this chapter or in others, should be determined on the basis of its clinical presentation and course as well as on the therapeutic considerations and priorities at the time of the consultation. Generally, if the sleep disorder is one of the major complaints and is perceived as a condition in itself, the present code should be used along with other pertinent diagnoses describing the psychopathology and pathophysiology involved in a given case. This category includes only those sleep disorders in which emotional causes are considered to be a primary factor, and which are not due to identifiable physical disorders classified elsewhere.

*Excludes:*   • sleep disorders (organic) (G47.–)

**F51.0  *Nonorganic insomnia***
A condition of unsatisfactory quantity and/or quality of sleep, which persists for a considerable period of time, including difficulty falling asleep, difficulty staying asleep, or early final wakening. Insomnia is a common symptom of many mental and physical disorders, and should be classified here in addition to the basic disorder only if it dominates the clinical picture.

*Excludes:*   • insomnia (organic) (G47.0)

**F51.1  *Nonorganic hypersomnia***
Hypersomnia is defined as a condition of either excessive daytime sleepiness and sleep attacks (not accounted for by an inadequate amount of sleep) or prolonged transition to the fully aroused state upon awakening. In the absence of an organic factor for the occurrence of hypersomnia, this condition is usually associated with mental disorders.

*Excludes:*   • hypersomnia (organic) (G47.1)
              • narcolepsy (G47.4)

**F51.2  *Nonorganic disorder of the sleep-wake schedule***
A lack of synchrony between the sleep-wake schedule and the desired sleep-wake schedule for the individual's environment, resulting in a complaint of either insomnia or hypersomnia.

Psychogenic inversion of:
• circadian ⎫
• nyctohemeral ⎬ rhythm
• sleep ⎭
*Excludes:*   • disorders of the sleep-wake schedule (organic) (G47.2)

### F51.3  Sleepwalking [somnambulism]

A state of altered consciousness in which phenomena of sleep and wakefulness are combined. During a sleepwalking episode the individual arises from bed, usually during the first third of nocturnal sleep, and walks about, exhibiting low levels of awareness, reactivity, and motor skill. Upon awakening, there is usually no recall of the event.

### F51.4  Sleep terrors [night terrors]

Nocturnal episodes of extreme terror and panic associated with intense vocalization, motility, and high levels of autonomic discharge. The individual sits up or gets up, usually during the first third of nocturnal sleep, with a panicky scream. Quite often he or she rushes to the door as if trying to escape, although very seldom leaves the room. Recall of the event, if any, is very limited (usually to one or two fragmentary mental images).

### F51.5  Nightmares

Dream experiences loaded with anxiety or fear. There is very detailed recall of the dream content. The dream experience is very vivid and usually includes themes involving threats to survival, security, or self-esteem. Quite often there is a recurrence of the same or similar frightening nightmare themes. During a typical episode there is a degree of autonomic discharge but no appreciable vocalization or body motility. Upon awakening the individual rapidly becomes alert and oriented.

Dream anxiety disorder

### F51.8  Other nonorganic sleep disorders

### F51.9  Nonorganic sleep disorder, unspecified

Emotional sleep disorder NOS

## F52    Sexual dysfunction, not caused by organic disorder or disease

Sexual dysfunction covers the various ways in which an individual is unable to participate in a sexual relationship as he or she would wish. Sexual response is a psychosomatic process and both psychological and somatic processes are usually involved in the causation of sexual dysfunction.

Excludes:  • Dhat syndrome (F48.8)

### F52.0  Lack or loss of sexual desire

Loss of sexual desire is the principal problem and is not secondary to other sexual difficulties, such as erectile failure or dyspareunia.

Frigidity
Hypoactive sexual desire disorder

*F52.1  Sexual aversion and lack of sexual enjoyment*
Either the prospect of sexual interaction produces sufficient fear or anxiety that
sexual activity is avoided (sexual aversion) or sexual responses occur normally
and orgasm is experienced but there is a lack of appropriate pleasure (lack of
sexual enjoyment).

Anhedonia (sexual)

*F52.2  Failure of genital response*
The principal problem in men is erectile dysfunction (difficulty in developing or
maintaining an erection suitable for satisfactory intercourse). In women, the
principal problem is vaginal dryness or failure of lubrication.

Female sexual arousal disorder
Male erectile disorder
Psychogenic impotence
*Excludes:* • impotence of organic origin (N48.4)

*F52.3  Orgasmic dysfunction*
Orgasm either does not occur or is markedly delayed.

Inhibited orgasm (male)(female)
Psychogenic anorgasmy

*F52.4  Premature ejaculation*
The inability to control ejaculation sufficiently for both partners to enjoy sexual
interaction.

*F52.5  Nonorganic vaginismus*
Spasm of the pelvic floor muscles that surround the vagina, causing occlusion of
the vaginal opening. Penile entry is either impossible or painful.
Psychogenic vaginismus
*Excludes:* • vaginismus (organic) (N94.2)

*F52.6  Nonorganic dyspareunia*
Dyspareunia (or pain during sexual intercourse) occurs in both women and men.
It can often be attributed to local pathology and should then properly be catego-
rized under the pathological condition. This category is to be used only if there is
no primary nonorganic sexual dysfunction (e.g. vaginismus or vaginal dryness).

Psychogenic dyspareunia
*Excludes:* • dyspareunia (organic) (N94.1)

*F52.7  Excessive sexual drive*
Nymphomania
Satyriasis

*F52.8  Other sexual dysfunction, not caused by organic disorder or disease*

*F52.9  Unspecified sexual dysfunction, not caused by organic disorder or disease*

**F53    Mental and behavioural disorders associated with the puerperium, not elsewhere classified**
This category includes only mental disorders associated with the puerperium (commencing within six weeks of delivery) that do not meet the criteria for disorders classified elsewhere in this chapter, either because insufficient information is available, or because it is considered that special additional clinical features are present that make their classification elsewhere inappropriate.

*F53.0  Mild mental and behavioural disorders associated with the puerperium, not elsewhere classified*
Depression:
• postnatal NOS
• postpartum NOS

*F53.1  Severe mental and behavioural disorders associated with the puerperium, not elsewhere classified*
Puerperal psychosis NOS

*F53.8  Other mental and behavioural disorders associated with the puerperium, not elsewhere classified*

*F53.9  Puerperal mental disorder, unspecified*

**F54    Psychological and behavioural factors associated with disorders or diseases classified elsewhere**
This category should be used to record the presence of psychological or behavioural influences thought to have played a major part in the etiology of physical disorders which can be classified to other chapters. Any resulting mental disturbances are usually mild, and often prolonged (such as worry, emotional conflict, apprehension) and do not of themselves justify the use of any of the categories in this chapter.

Psychological factors affecting physical conditions
Examples of the use of this category are:
• asthma F54 and J45.–
• dermatitis F54 and L23–L25
• gastric ulcer F54 and K25.–
• mucous colitis F54 and K58.–
• ulcerative colitis F54 and K51.–
• urticaria F54 and L50.–

Use additional code, if desired, to identify the associated physical disorder.

*Excludes:* • tension-type headache (G44.2)

**F55    *Abuse of non-dependence-producing substances***
A wide variety of medicaments and folk remedies may be involved, but the particularly important groups are: (a) psychotropic drugs that do not produce dependence, such as antidepressants, (b) laxatives, and (c) analgesics that may be purchased without medical prescription, such as aspirin and paracetamol.

Persistent use of these substances often involves unnecessary contacts with medical professionals or supporting staff, and is sometimes accompanied by harmful physical effects of the substances. Attempts to dissuade or forbid the use of the substance are often met with resistance; for laxatives and analgesics this may be in spite of warnings about (or even the development of) physical harm such as renal dysfunction or electrolyte disturbances. Although it is usually clear that the patient has a strong motivation to take the substance, dependence or withdrawal symptoms do not develop as in the case of the psychoactive substances specified in F10–F19.

Abuse of:
• antacids
• herbal or folk remedies
• steroids or hormones
• vitamins
Laxative habit
*Excludes:* • abuse of psychoactive substances (F10–F19)

**F59    *Unspecified behavioural syndromes associated with physiological disturbances and physical factors***
Psychogenic physiological dysfunction NOS

**Disorders of adult personality and behaviour
(F60–F69)**

This section includes a variety of conditions and behaviour patterns of clinical significance which tend to be persistent and appear to be the expression of the individual's characteristic lifestyle and mode of relating to himself or herself and others. Some of these conditions and patterns of behaviour emerge early in the course of individual development, as a result of both constitutional factors and social experience, while others are acquired later in life. Specific personality disorders (F60.–), mixed and other personality disorders (F61.–), and enduring personality changes (F62.–) are deeply ingrained and enduring behaviour patterns, manifesting as inflexible responses to a broad range of personal and social situations. They represent extreme or significant deviations from the way in which the average individual in a given culture perceives, thinks, feels and, particularly, relates to others. Such behaviour patterns tend to be stable and to encompass multiple domains of behaviour and psychological functioning. They are frequently, but not always, associated with various degrees of subjective distress and problems of social performance.

**F60**    *Specific personality disorders*
These are severe disturbances in the personality and behavioural tendencies of the individual; not directly resulting from disease, damage, or other insult to the brain, or from another psychiatric disorder; usually involving several areas of the personality; nearly always associated with considerable personal distress and social disruption; and usually manifest since childhood or adolescence and continuing throughout adulthood.

*F60.0  Paranoid personality disorder*
Personality disorder characterized by excessive sensitivity to setbacks, unforgiveness of insults; suspiciousness and a tendency to distort experience by misconstruing the neutral or friendly actions of others as hostile or contemptuous; recurrent suspicions, without justification, regarding the sexual fidelity of the spouse or sexual partner; and a combative and tenacious sense of personal rights. There may be excessive self-importance, and there is often excessive self-reference.

Personality (disorder):
• expansive paranoid
• fanatic
• querulant
• paranoid
• sensitive paranoid
*Excludes:* • paranoia (F22.0)
           • querulans (F22.8)
           paranoid:
           • psychosis (F22.0)
           • schizophrenia (F20.0)
           • state (F22.0)

*F60.1  Schizoid personality disorder*
Personality disorder characterized by withdrawal from affectional, social and other contacts with preference for fantasy, solitary activities, and introspection. There is a limited capacity to express feelings and to experience pleasure.

*Excludes:* • Asperger's syndrome (F84.5)
           • delusional disorder (F22.0)
           • schizoid disorder of childhood (F84.5)
           • schizophrenia (F20.–)
           • schizotypal disorder (F21)

### F60.2 Dissocial personality disorder

Personality disorder characterized by disregard for social obligations, and callous unconcern for the feelings of others. There is gross disparity between behaviour and the prevailing social norms. Behaviour is not readily modifiable by adverse experience, including punishment. There is a low tolerance to frustration and a low threshold for discharge of aggression, including violence; there is a tendency to blame others, or to offer plausible rationalizations for the behaviour bringing the patient into conflict with society.

Personality (disorder):
- amoral
- antisocial
- asocial
- psychopathic
- sociopathic

Excludes:  • conduct disorders (F91.–)
            • emotionally unstable personality disorder (F60.3)

### F60.3 Emotionally unstable personality disorder

Personality disorder characterized by a definite tendency to act impulsively and without consideration of the consequences; the mood is unpredictable and capricious. There is a liability to outbursts of emotion and an incapacity to control the behavioural explosions. There is a tendency to quarrelsome behaviour and to conflicts with others, especially when impulsive acts are thwarted or censored. Two types may be distinguished: the impulsive type, characterized predominantly by emotional instability and lack of impulse control, and the borderline type, characterized in addition by disturbances in self-image, aims, and internal preferences, by chronic feelings of emptiness, by intense and unstable interpersonal relationships, and by a tendency to self-destructive behaviour, including suicide gestures and attempts.

Personality (disorder):
- aggressive
- borderline
- explosive

Excludes:  • dissocial personality disorder (F60.2)

### F60.4 Histrionic personality disorder

Personality disorder characterized by shallow and labile affectivity, self-dramatization, theatricality, exaggerated expression of emotions, suggestibility, egocentricity, self-indulgence, lack of consideration for others, easily hurt feelings, and continuous seeking for appreciation, excitement and attention.

Personality (disorder):
- hysterical
- psychoinfantile

### F60.5 Anankastic personality disorder

Personality disorder characterized by feelings of doubt, perfectionism, excessive conscientiousness, checking and preoccupation with details, stubbornness, caution, and rigidity. There may be insistent and unwelcome thoughts or impulses that do not attain the severity of an obsessive-compulsive disorder.

Personality (disorder):
- compulsive
- obsessional
- obsessive-compulsive

*Excludes:* • obsessive-compulsive disorder (F42.–)

### F60.6 Anxious [avoidant] personality disorder

Personality disorder characterized by feelings of tension and apprehension, insecurity and inferiority. There is a continuous yearning to be liked and accepted, a hypersensitivity to rejection and criticism with restricted personal attachments, and a tendency to avoid certain activities by habitual exaggeration of the potential dangers or risks in everyday situations.

### F60.7 Dependent personality disorder

Personality disorder characterized by pervasive passive reliance on other people to make one's major and minor life decisions, great fear of abandonment, feelings of helplessness and incompetence, passive compliance with the wishes of elders and others, and a weak response to the demands of daily life. Lack of vigour may show itself in the intellectual or emotional spheres; there is often a tendency to transfer responsibility to others.

Personality (disorder):
- asthenic
- inadequate
- passive
- self-defeating

### F60.8 Other specific personality disorders

Personality (disorder):
- eccentric
- 'haltlose' type
- immature
- narcissistic
- passive-aggressive
- psychoneurotic

### F60.9 Personality disorder, unspecified

Character neurosis NOS
Pathological personality NOS

### F61    *Mixed and other personality disorders*

This category is intended for personality disorders that are often troublesome but do not demonstrate the specific pattern of symptoms that characterize the disorders described in F60.–. As a result they are often more difficult to diagnose than the disorders in F60.–.

Examples include:

- Mixed personality disorders with features of several of the disorders in F60.– but without a predominant set of symptoms that would allow a more specific diagnosis
- troublesome personality changes, not classifiable to F60.– or F62.–, and regarded as secondary to a main diagnosis of a coexisting affective or anxiety disorder.

*Excludes:*  • accentuated personality traits (Z73.1)

### F62    *Enduring personality changes, not attributable to brain damage and disease*

Disorders of adult personality and behaviour that have developed in persons with no previous personality disorder following exposure to catastrophic or excessive prolonged stress, or following a severe psychiatric illness. These diagnoses should be made only when there is evidence of a definite and enduring change in a person's pattern of perceiving, relating to, or thinking about the environment and himself or herself. The personality change should be significant and be associated with inflexible and maladaptive behaviour not present before the pathogenic experience. The change should not be a direct manifestation of another mental disorder or a residual symptom of any antecedent mental disorder.

*Excludes:*  • personality and behavioural disorder due to brain disease, damage and dysfunction (F07.–)

#### F62.0 *Enduring personality change after catastrophic experience*

Enduring personality change, present for at least two years, following exposure to catastrophic stress. The stress must be so extreme that it is not necessary to consider personal vulnerability in order to explain its profound effect on the personality. The disorder is characterized by a hostile or distrustful attitude toward the world, social withdrawal, feelings of emptiness or hopelessness, a chronic feeling of "being on edge" as if constantly threatened, and estrangement. Posttraumatic stress disorder (F43.1) may precede this type of personality change.

Personality change after:

- concentration camp experiences
- disasters
- prolonged:
    - captivity with an imminent possibility of being killed
    - exposure to life-threatening situations such as being a victim of terrorism

• torture

*Excludes:* • post-traumatic stress disorder (F43.1)

### F62.1 Enduring personality change after psychiatric illness

Personality change, persisting for at least two years, attributable to the traumatic experience of suffering from a severe psychiatric illness. The change cannot be explained by a previous personality disorder and should be differentiated from residual schizophrenia and other states of incomplete recovery from an antecedent mental disorder. This disorder is characterized by an excessive dependence on and a demanding attitude towards others; conviction of being changed or stigmatized by the illness, leading to an inability to form and maintain close and confiding personal relationships and to social isolation; passivity, reduced interests, and diminished involvement in leisure activities; persistent complaints of being ill, which may be associated with hypochondriacal claims and illness behaviour; dysphoric or labile mood, not due to the presence of a current mental disorder or antecedent mental disorder with residual affective symptoms; and longstanding problems in social and occupational functioning.

### F62.8 Other enduring personality changes

Chronic pain personality syndrome

### F62.9 Enduring personality change, unspecified

## F63  Habit and impulse disorders

This category includes certain disorders of behaviour that are not classifiable under other categories. They are characterized by repeated acts that have no clear rational motivation, cannot be controlled, and generally harm the patient's own interests and those of other people. The patient reports that the behaviour is associated with impulses to action. The cause of these disorders is not understood and they are grouped together because of broad descriptive similarities, not because they are known to share any other important features.

*Excludes:* • habitual excessive use of alcohol or psychoactive substances (F10–F19)

• impulse and habit disorders involving sexual behaviour (F65.–)

### 63.0 Pathological gambling

The disorder consists of frequent, repeated episodes of gambling that dominate the patient's life to the detriment of social, occupational, material, and family values and commitments.

Compulsive gambling

*Excludes:* • excessive gambling by manic patients (F30.–)

• gambling and betting NOS (Z72.6)

• gambling in dissocial personality disorder (F60.2)

### F63.1  Pathological fire-setting [pyromania]

Disorder characterized by multiple acts of, or attempts at, setting fire to property or other objects, without apparent motive, and by a persistent preoccupation with subjects related to fire and burning. This behaviour is often associated with feelings of increasing tension before the act, and intense excitement immediately afterwards.

Excludes:  fire-setting (by)(in):
- adult with dissocial personality disorder (F60.2)
- alcohol or psychoactive substance intoxication (F10–F19, with common fourth character .0)
- as the reason for observation for suspected mental disorder (Z03.2)
- conduct disorders (F91.–)
- organic mental disorders (F00–F09)
- schizophrenia (F20.–)

### F63.2  Pathological stealing [kleptomania]

Disorder characterized by repeated failure to resist impulses to steal objects that are not acquired for personal use or monetary gain. The objects may instead be discarded, given away, or hoarded. This behaviour is usually accompanied by an increasing sense of tension before, and a sense of gratification during and immediately after, the act.

Excludes:  • depressive disorder with stealing (F31–F33)
- organic mental disorders (F00–F09)
- shoplifting as the reason for observation for suspected mental disorder (Z03.2)

### F63.3  Trichotillomania

A disorder characterized by noticeable hair-loss due to a recurrent failure to resist impulses to pull out hairs. The hair-pulling is usually preceded by mounting tension and is followed by a sense of relief or gratification. This diagnosis should not be made if there is a pre-existing inflammation of the skin, or if the hair-pulling is in response to a delusion or a hallucination.

Excludes:  • stereotyped movement disorder with hair-plucking (F98.4)

### F63.8  Other habit and impulse disorders

Other kinds of persistently repeated maladaptive behaviour that are not secondary to a recognized psychiatric syndrome, and in which it appears that the patient is repeatedly failing to resist impulses to carry out the behaviour. There is a prodromal period of tension with a feeling of release at the time of the act.

Intermittent explosive disorder

*F63.9 Habit and impulse disorder, unspecified*

## F64    Gender identity disorders

### F64.0 Transsexualism

A desire to live and be accepted as a member of the opposite sex, usually accompanied by a sense of discomfort with, or inappropriateness of, one's anatomic sex, and a wish to have surgery and hormonal treatment to make one's body as congruent as possible with one's preferred sex.

### F64.1 Dual-role transvestism

The wearing of clothes of the opposite sex for part of the individual's existence in order to enjoy the temporary experience of membership of the opposite sex, but without any desire for a more permanent sex change or associated surgical reassignment, and without sexual excitement accompanying the cross-dressing.

Gender identity disorder of adolescence or adulthood, nontranssexual type
*Excludes:* • fetishistic transvestism (F65.1)

### F64.2 Gender identity disorder of childhood

A disorder, usually first manifest during early childhood (and always well before puberty), characterized by a persistent and intense distress about assigned sex, together with a desire to be (or insistence that one is) of the other sex. There is a persistent preoccupation with the dress and activities of the opposite sex and repudiation of the individual's own sex. The diagnosis requires a profound disturbance of the normal gender identity; mere tomboyishness in girls or girlish behaviour in boys is not sufficient. Gender identity disorders in individuals who have reached or are entering puberty should not be classified here but in F66.–.

*Excludes:* • egodystonic sexual orientation (F66.1)
           • sexual maturation disorder (F66.0)

### F64.8 Other gender identity disorders

### F64.9 Gender identity disorder, unspecified
• Gender-role disorder NOS

## F65    Disorders of sexual preference
*Includes:* • paraphilias

### F65.0 Fetishism

Reliance on some non-living object as a stimulus for sexual arousal and sexual gratification. Many fetishes are extensions of the human body, such as articles of clothing or footwear. Other common examples are characterized by some particular texture such as rubber, plastic or leather. Fetish objects vary in their importance to the individual. In some cases they simply serve to enhance sexual excitement achieved in ordinary ways (e.g. having the partner wear a particular garment).

### F65.1 Fetishistic transvestism
The wearing of clothes of the opposite sex principally to obtain sexual excitement and to create the appearance of a person of the opposite sex. Fetishistic transvestism is distinguished from transsexual transvestism by its clear association with sexual arousal and the strong desire to remove the clothing once orgasm occurs and sexual arousal declines. It can occur as an earlier phase in the development of transsexualism.

Transvestic fetishism

### F65.2 Exhibitionism
A recurrent or persistent tendency to expose the genitalia to strangers (usually of the opposite sex) or to people in public places, without inviting or intending closer contact. There is usually, but not invariably, sexual excitement at the time of the exposure and the act is commonly followed by masturbation.

### F65.3 Voyeurism
A recurrent or persistent tendency to look at people engaging in sexual or intimate behaviour such as undressing. This is carried out without the observed people being aware, and usually leads to sexual excitement and masturbation.

### F65.4 Paedophilia
A sexual preference for children, boys or girls or both, usually of prepubertal or early pubertal age.

### F65.5 Sadomasochism
A preference for sexual activity which involves the infliction of pain or humiliation, or bondage. If the subject prefers to be the recipient of such stimulation this is called masochism; if the provider, sadism. Often an individual obtains sexual excitement from both sadistic and masochistic activities.

Masochism
Sadism

### F65.6 Multiple disorders of sexual preference
Sometimes more than one abnormal sexual preference occurs in one person and there is none of first rank. The most common combination is fetishism, transvestism and sadomasochism.

### F65.8 Other disorders of sexual preference
A variety of other patterns of sexual preference and activity, including making obscene telephone calls, rubbing up against people for sexual stimulation in

crowded public places, sexual activity with animals, and use of strangulation or anoxia for intensifying sexual excitement.

Frotteurism
Necrophilia

#### F65.9 Disorder of sexual preference, unspecified
Sexual deviation NOS

### F66 Psychological and behavioural disorders associated with sexual development and orientation
*Note:* Sexual orientation by itself is not to be regarded as a disorder.

#### F66.0 Sexual maturation disorder
The patient suffers from uncertainty about his or her gender identity or sexual orientation, which causes anxiety or depression. Most commonly this occurs in adolescents who are not certain whether they are homosexual, heterosexual or bisexual in orientation, or in individuals who, after a period of apparently stable sexual orientation (often within a longstanding relationship), find that their sexual orientation is changing.

#### F66.1 Egodystonic sexual orientation
The gender identity or sexual preference (heterosexual, homosexual, bisexual, or prepubertal) is not in doubt, but the individual wishes it were different because of associated psychological and behavioural disorders, and may seek treatment in order to change it.

#### F66.2 Sexual relationship disorder
The gender identity or sexual orientation (heterosexual, homosexual, or bisexual) is responsible for difficulties in forming or maintaining a relationship with a sexual partner.

#### F66.8 Other psychosexual development disorders

#### F66.9 Psychosexual development disorder, unspecified

### F68 Other disorders of adult personality and behaviour

#### F68.0 Elaboration of physical symptoms for psychological reasons
Physical symptoms compatible with and originally due to a confirmed physical disorder, disease or disability become exaggerated or prolonged due to the psychological state of the patient. The patient is commonly distressed by this pain or disability, and is often preoccupied with worries, which may be justified, of the possibility of prolonged or progressive disability or pain.

Compensation neurosis

*F68.1  Intentional production or feigning of symptoms or disabilities, either physical or psychological [factitious disorder]*

The patient feigns symptoms repeatedly for no obvious reason and may even inflict self-harm in order to produce symptoms or signs. The motivation is obscure and presumably internal with the aim of adopting the sick role. The disorder is often combined with marked disorders of personality and relationships.

Hospital hopper syndrome
Münchhausen's syndrome
Peregrinating patient
*Excludes:*  • factitial dermatitis (L98.1)
          • person feigning illness (with obvious motivation) (Z76.5)

*F68.8  Other specified disorders of adult personality and behaviour*
Character disorder NOS
Relationship disorder NOS

**F69**   *Unspecified disorder of adult personality and behaviour*

## Mental retardation
## (F70–F79)

A condition of arrested or incomplete development of the mind, which is especially characterized by impairment of skills manifested during the developmental period, skills which contribute to the overall level of intelligence, i.e. cognitive, language, motor, and social abilities. Retardation can occur with or without any other mental or physical condition.

Degrees of mental retardation are conventionally estimated by standardized intelligence tests. These can be supplemented by scales assessing social adaptation in a given environment. These measures provide an approximate indication of the degree of mental retardation. The diagnosis will also depend on the overall assessment of intellectual functioning by a skilled diagnostician.

Intellectual abilities and social adaptation may change over time, and, however poor, may improve as a result of training and rehabilitation. Diagnosis should be based on the current levels of functioning.

The following fourth-character subdivisions are for use with categories F70–F79 to identify the extent of impairment of behaviour:

*.0  With the statement of no, or minimal, impairment of behaviour*

*.1  Significant impairment of behaviour requiring attention or treatment*

*.8  Other impairments of behaviour*

*.9 Without mention of impairment of behaviour*
Use additional code, if desired, to identify associated conditions such as autism, other developmental disorders, epilepsy, conduct disorders, or severe physical handicap.

**F70    *Mild mental retardation***
Approximate IQ range of 50 to 69 (in adults, mental age from 9 to under 12 years). Likely to result in some learning difficulties in school. Many adults will be able to work and maintain good social relationships and contribute to society.

*Includes:*   • feeble-mindedness
          • mild mental subnormality

**F71    *Moderate mental retardation***
Approximate IQ range of 35 to 49 (in adults, mental age from 6 to under 9 years). Likely to result in marked developmental delays in childhood but most can learn to develop some degree of independence in self-care and acquire adequate communication and academic skills. Adults will need varying degrees of support to live and work in the community.

*Includes:*   • moderate mental subnormality

**F72    *Severe mental retardation***
Approximate IQ range of 20 to 34 (in adults, mental age from 3 to under 6 years). Likely to result in continuous need of support.

*Includes:*   • severe mental subnormality

**F73    *Profound mental retardation***
IQ under 20 (in adults, mental age below 3 years). Results in severe limitation in self-care, continence, communication and mobility.

*Includes:*   • profound mental subnormality

**F78    *Other mental retardation***

**F79    *Unspecified mental retardation***
*Includes:*   • mental:
          • deficiency NOS
          • subnormality NOS

**Disorders of psychological development**
**(F80–F89)**

The disorders included in this section have in common: (a) onset invariably during infancy or childhood; (b) impairment or delay in development of functions that are strongly related to biological maturation of the central nervous system; and (c) a steady course without remissions and relapses. In most cases, the functions affected include language, visuo-spatial skills, and motor coordination. Usually, the delay or impairment has been present from as early as it could be detected reliably and will diminish progressively as the child grows older, although milder deficits often remain in adult life.

**F80     Specific developmental disorders of speech and language**
Disorders in which normal patterns of language acquisition are disturbed from the early stages of development. The conditions are not directly attributable to neurological or speech mechanism abnormalities, sensory impairments, mental retardation, or environmental factors. Specific developmental disorders of speech and language are often followed by associated problems, such as difficulties in reading and spelling, abnormalities in interpersonal relationships, and emotional and behavioural disorders.

**F80.0  Specific speech articulation disorder**
A specific developmental disorder in which the child's use of speech sounds is below the appropriate level for its mental age, but in which there is a normal level of language skills.

Developmental:
• phonological disorder
• speech articulation disorder
Dyslalia
Functional speech articulation disorder
Lalling
*Excludes:*  speech articulation impairment (due to):
            • aphasia NOS (R47.0)
            • apraxia (R48.2)
            • hearing loss (H90–H91)
            • mental retardation (F70–F79)
            • with language developmental disorder:
              • expressive (80.1)
              • receptive (F80.2)

**F80.1  Expressive language disorder**
A specific developmental disorder in which the child's ability to use expressive spoken language is markedly below the appropriate level for its mental age, but in which language comprehension is within normal limits. There may or may not be abnormalities in articulation.

Developmental dysphasia or aphasia, expressive type
*Excludes:*  • acquired aphasia with epilepsy [Landau-Kleffner] (F80.3)

- developmental dysphasia or aphasia, receptive type (F80.2)
- dysphasia and aphasia NOS (R47.0)
- elective mutism (F94.0)
- mental retardation (F70–F79)
- pervasive developmental disorders (F84.–)

### F80.2  Receptive language disorder

A specific developmental disorder in which the child's understanding of language is below the appropriate level for its mental age. In virtually all cases expressive language will also be markedly affected and abnormalities in word-sound production are common.

Congenital auditory imperception
Developmental:
- dysphasia or aphasia, receptive type
- Wernicke's aphasia
Word deafness

Excludes:  • acquired aphasia with epilepsy [Landau–Kleffner] (F80.3)
            autism (F84.0–F84.1)
            dysphasia and aphasia:
            • NOS (R47.0)
            • expressive type (F80.1)
            elective mutism (F94.0)
            language delay due to deafness (H90–H91)
            mental retardation (F70–F79)

### F80.3  Acquired aphasia with epilepsy [Landau–Kleffner]

A disorder in which the child, having previously made normal progress in language development, loses both receptive and expressive language skills but retains general intelligence; the onset of the disorder is accompanied by paroxysmal abnormalities on the EEG, and in the majority of cases also by epileptic seizures. Usually the onset is between the ages of three and seven years, with skills being lost over days or weeks. The temporal association between the onset of seizures and loss of language is variable, with one preceding the other (either way round) by a few months to two years. An inflammatory encephalitic process has been suggested as a possible cause of this disorder. About two-thirds of patients are left with a more or less severe receptive language deficit.

Excludes:  • aphasia (due to):
            • NOS (R47.0)
            • autism (F84.0–F84.1)
            • disintegrative disorders of childhood (F84.2–F84.3)

### F80.8  Other developmental disorders of speech and language
Lisping

*F80.9  Developmental disorder of speech and language, unspecified*

Language disorder NOS

*F81  Specific developmental disorders of scholastic skills*

Disorders in which the normal patterns of skill acquisition are disturbed from the early stages of development. This is not simply a consequence of a lack of opportunity to learn, it is not solely a result of mental retardation, and it is not due to any form of acquired brain trauma or disease.

*F81.0  Specific reading disorder*

The main feature is a specific and significant impairment in the development of reading skills that is not solely accounted for by mental age, visual acuity problems, or inadequate schooling. Reading comprehension skill, reading word recognition, oral reading skill, and performance of tasks requiring reading may all be affected. Spelling difficulties are frequently associated with specific reading disorder and often remain into adolescence even after some progress in reading has been made. Specific developmental disorders of reading are commonly preceded by a history of disorders in speech or language development. Associated emotional and behavioural disturbances are common during the school age period.

'Backward reading'

Developmental dyslexia

Specific reading retardation

*Excludes:*   • alexia NOS (R48.0)

           • dyslexia NOS (R48.0)

           • reading difficulties secondary to emotional disorders (F93.–)

*F81.1  Specific spelling disorder*

The main feature is a specific and significant impairment in the development of spelling skills in the absence of a history of specific reading disorder, which is not solely accounted for by low mental age, visual acuity problems, or inadequate schooling. The ability to spell orally and to write out words correctly are both affected.

Specific spelling retardation (without reading disorder)

*Excludes:*   • agraphia NOS (R48.8)

           spelling difficulties:

           • associated with a reading disorder (F81.0)

           • due to inadequate teaching (Z55.8)

*F81.2  Specific disorder of arithmetical skills*

Involves a specific impairment in arithmetical skills that is not solely explicable on the basis of general mental retardation or of inadequate schooling. The deficit concerns mastery of basic computational skills of addition, subtraction, multiplication, and division rather than of the more abstract mathematical skills involved in algebra, trigonometry, geometry, or calculus.

Developmental:
- acalculia
- arithmetical disorder
- Gerstmann's syndrome

*Excludes:*   •  acalculia NOS (R48.8)
        arithmetical difficulties:
        •  associated with a reading or spelling disorder (F81.3)
        •  due to inadequate teaching (Z55.8)

### F81.3  Mixed disorder of scholastic skills
An ill-defined residual category of disorders in which both arithmetical and reading or spelling skills are significantly impaired, but in which the disorder is not solely explicable in terms of general mental retardation or of inadequate schooling. It should be used for disorders meeting the criteria for both F81.2 and either F81.0 or F81.1.

*Excludes:*   specific:
        •  disorder of arithmetical skills (F81.2)
        •  reading disorder (F81.0)
        •  spelling disorder (F81.1)

### F81.8  Other developmental disorders of scholastic skills
Developmental expressive writing disorder

### F81.9  Developmental disorder of scholastic skills, unspecified
Knowledge acquisition disability NOS
Learning:
- disability NOS
- disorder NOS

### F82    Specific developmental disorder of motor function
A disorder in which the main feature is a serious impairment in the development of motor coordination that is not solely explicable in terms of general intellectual retardation or of any specific congenital or acquired neurological disorder. Nevertheless, in most cases a careful clinical examination shows marked neurodevelopmental immaturities such as choreiform movements of unsupported limbs or mirror movements and other associated motor features, as well as signs of impaired fine and gross motor coordination.

Clumsy child syndrome
Developmental:
- coordination disorder
- dyspraxia

*Excludes:*  • abnormalities of gait and mobility (R26.–)
            lack of coordination (R27.–)
          • secondary to mental retardation (F70–F79)

**F83   *Mixed specific developmental disorders***
A residual category for disorders in which there is some admixture of specific developmental disorders of speech and language, of scholastic skills, and of motor function, but in which none predominates sufficiently to constitute the prime diagnosis. This mixed category should be used only when there is a major overlap between each of these specific developmental disorders. The disorders are usually, but not always, associated with some degree of general impairment of cognitive functions. Thus, the category should be used when there are dysfunctions meeting the criteria for two or more of F80.–, F81.– and F82.

**F84   *Pervasive developmental disorders***
A group of disorders characterized by qualitative abnormalities in reciprocal social interactions and in patterns of communication, and by a restricted, stereotyped, repetitive repertoire of interests and activities. These qualitative abnormalities are a pervasive feature of the individual's functioning in all situations.
  Use additional code, if desired, to identify any associated medical condition and mental retardation.

***F84.0  Childhood autism***
A type of pervasive developmental disorder that is defined by: (a) the presence of abnormal or impaired development that is manifest before the age of three years, and (b) the characteristic type of abnormal functioning in all the three areas of psychopathology: reciprocal social interaction, communication, and restricted, stereotyped, repetitive behaviour. In addition to these specific diagnostic features, a range of other nonspecific problems are common, such as phobias, sleeping and eating disturbances, temper tantrums, and (self-directed) aggression.

Autistic disorder
Infantile:
• autism
• psychosis
Kanner's syndrome
*Excludes:*  • autistic psychopathy (F84.5)

***F84.1  Atypical autism***
A type of pervasive developmental disorder that differs from childhood autism either in age of onset or in failing to fulfil all three sets of diagnostic criteria. This subcategory should be used when there is abnormal and impaired development that is present only after age three years, and a lack of sufficient demonstrable abnormalities in one or two of the three areas of psychopathology required

for the diagnosis of autism (namely, reciprocal social interactions, communication, and restricted, stereotyped, repetitive behaviour) in spite of characteristic abnormalities in the other area(s). Atypical autism arises most often in profoundly retarded individuals and in individuals with a severe specific developmental disorder of receptive language.

Atypical childhood psychosis
Mental retardation with autistic features

Use additional code (F70–F79), if desired, to identify mental retardation.

### F84.2  Rett's syndrome
A condition, so far found only in girls, in which apparently normal early development is followed by partial or complete loss of speech and of skills in locomotion and use of hands, together with deceleration in head growth, usually with an onset between seven and 24 months of age. Loss of purposive hand movements, hand-wringing stereotypies, and hyperventilation are characteristic. Social and play development are arrested but social interest tends to be maintained. Trunk ataxia and apraxia start to develop by age four years and choreoathetoid movements frequently follow. Severe mental retardation almost invariably results.

### F84.3  Other childhood disintegrative disorder
A type of pervasive developmental disorder that is defined by a period of entirely normal development before the onset of the disorder, followed by a definite loss of previously acquired skills in several areas of development over the course of a few months. Typically, this is accompanied by a general loss of interest in the environment, by stereotyped, repetitive motor mannerisms, and by autistic-like abnormalities in social interaction and communication. In some cases the disorder can be shown to be due to some associated encephalopathy but the diagnosis should be made on the behavioural features.

Dementia infantilis
Disintegrative psychosis
Heller's syndrome
Symbiotic psychosis
Use additional code, if desired, to identify any associated neurological condition.
*Excludes:* • Rett's syndrome (F84.2)

### F84.4  Overactive disorder associated with mental retardation and stereotyped movements
An ill-defined disorder of uncertain nosological validity. The category is designed to include a group of children with severe mental retardation (IQ below 50) who show major problems in hyperactivity and in attention, as well as stereotyped behaviours. They tend not to benefit from stimulant drugs (unlike

those with an IQ in the normal range) and may exhibit a severe dysphoric reaction (sometimes with psychomotor retardation) when given stimulants. In adolescence, the overactivity tends to be replaced by underactivity (a pattern that is not usual in hyperkinetic children with normal intelligence). This syndrome is also often associated with a variety of developmental delays, either specific or global. The extent to which the behavioural pattern is a function of low IQ or of organic brain damage is not known.

### F84.5 Asperger's syndrome
A disorder of uncertain nosological validity, characterized by the same type of qualitative abnormalities of reciprocal social interaction that typify autism, together with a restricted, stereotyped, repetitive repertoire of interests and activities. It differs from autism primarily in the fact that there is no general delay or retardation in language or in cognitive development. This disorder is often associated with marked clumsiness. There is a strong tendency for the abnormalities to persist into adolescence and adult life. Psychotic episodes occasionally occur in early adult life.

Autistic psychopathy
Schizoid disorder of childhood

### F84.8 Other pervasive developmental disorders

### F84.9 Pervasive developmental disorder, unspecified

## F88 Other disorders of psychological development
Developmental agnosia

## F89 Unspecified disorder of psychological development
Developmental disorder NOS

## Behavioural and emotional disorders with onset usually occurring in childhood and adolescence
## (F90–F98)

## F90 Hyperkinetic disorders
A group of disorders characterized by an early onset (usually in the first five years of life), lack of persistence in activities that require cognitive involvement, and a tendency to move from one activity to another without completing any one, together with disorganized, ill-regulated, and excessive activity. Several other abnormalities may be associated. Hyperkinetic children are often reckless and impulsive, prone to accidents, and find themselves in disciplinary trouble because of unthinking breaches of rules rather than deliberate defiance. Their

relationships with adults are often socially disinhibited, with a lack of normal caution and reserve. They are unpopular with other children and may become isolated. Impairment of cognitive functions is common, and specific delays in motor and language development are disproportionately frequent. Secondary complications include dissocial behaviour and low self-esteem.

*Excludes:* • anxiety disorders (F41.–)
• mood [affective] disorders (F30–F39)
• pervasive developmental disorders (F84.–)
• schizophrenia (F20.–)

### F90.0 Disturbance of activity and attention
Attention deficit:
• disorder with hyperactivity
• hyperactivity disorder
• syndrome with hyperactivity
*Excludes:* • hyperkinetic disorder associated with conduct disorder (F90.1)

### F90.1 Hyperkinetic conduct disorder
Hyperkinetic disorder associated with conduct disorder

### F90.8 Other hyperkinetic disorders

### F90.9 Hyperkinetic disorder, unspecified
Hyperkinetic reaction of childhood or adolescence NOS
Hyperkinetic syndrome NOS

## F91  Conduct disorders
Disorders characterized by a repetitive and persistent pattern of dissocial, aggressive, or defiant conduct. Such behaviour should amount to major violations of age-appropriate social expectations; it should therefore be more severe than ordinary childish mischief or adolescent rebelliousness and should imply an enduring pattern of behaviour (six months or longer). Features of conduct disorder can also be symptomatic of other psychiatric conditions, in which case the underlying diagnosis should be preferred.

Examples of the behaviours on which the diagnosis is based include excessive levels of fighting or bullying, cruelty to other people or animals, severe destructiveness to property, fire-setting, stealing, repeated lying, truancy from school and running away from home, unusually frequent and severe temper tantrums, and disobedience. Any one of these behaviours, if marked, is sufficient for the diagnosis, but isolated dissocial acts are not.

*Excludes:* • mood [affective] (F30–F39)
pervasive developmental disorders (F84.–)

schizophrenia (F20.–)

when associated with:

- emotional disorders (F92.–)
- hyperkinetic disorders (F90.1)

### F91.0  Conduct disorder confined to the family context

Conduct disorder involving dissocial or aggressive behaviour (and not merely oppositional, defiant, disruptive behaviour), in which the abnormal behaviour is entirely, or almost entirely, confined to the home and to interactions with members of the nuclear family or immediate household. The disorder requires that the overall criteria for F91.– be met; even severely disturbed parent–child relationships are not of themselves sufficient for diagnosis.

### F91.1  Unsocialized conduct disorder

Disorder characterized by the combination of persistent dissocial or aggressive behaviour (meeting the overall criteria for F91.– and not merely comprising oppositional, defiant, disruptive behaviour) with significant pervasive abnormalities in the individual's relationships with other children.

Conduct disorder, solitary aggressive type
Unsocialized aggressive disorder

### F91.2  Socialized conduct disorder

Disorder involving persistent dissocial or aggressive behaviour (meeting the overall criteria for F91.– and not merely comprising oppositional, defiant, disruptive behaviour) occurring in individuals who are generally well integrated into their peer group.

Conduct disorder, group type
Group delinquency
Offences in the context of gang membership
Stealing in company with others
Truancy from school

### F91.3  Oppositional defiant disorder

Conduct disorder, usually occurring in younger children, primarily characterized by markedly defiant, disobedient, disruptive behaviour that does not include delinquent acts or the more extreme forms of aggressive or dissocial behaviour. The disorder requires that the overall criteria for F91.– be met; even severely mischievous or naughty behaviour is not in itself sufficient for diagnosis. Caution should be employed before using this category, especially with older children, because clinically significant conduct disorder will usually be accompanied by dissocial or aggressive behaviour that goes beyond mere defiance, disobedience, or disruptiveness.

*F91.8  Other conduct disorders*

*F91.9  Conduct disorder, unspecified*
Childhood:
• behavioural disorder NOS
• conduct disorder NOS

**F92    Mixed disorders of conduct and emotions**
A group of disorders characterized by the combination of persistently aggressive, dissocial or defiant behaviour with overt and marked symptoms of
depression, anxiety or other emotional upsets. The criteria for both conduct
disorders of childhood (F91.–) and emotional disorders of childhood (F93.–) or
an adult-type neurotic diagnosis (F40–F48) or a mood disorder (F30–F39)
must be met.

*F92.0  Depressive conduct disorder*
This category requires the combination of conduct disorder (F91.–) with persistent and marked depression of mood (F32.–), as demonstrated by symptoms
such as excessive misery, loss of interest and pleasure in usual activities, self-
blame, and hopelessness; disturbances of sleep or appetite may also be present.

Conduct disorder in F91.– associated with depressive disorder in F32.–

*F92.8  Other mixed disorders of conduct and emotions*
This category requires the combination of conduct disorder (F91.–) with persistent and marked emotional symptoms such as anxiety, obsessions or compul-
sions, depersonalization or derealization, phobias, or hypochondriasis.

Conduct disorder in F91.– associated with:
• emotional disorder in F93.–
• neurotic disorder in F40–F48

*F92.9  Mixed disorder of conduct and emotions, unspecified*

**F93    Emotional disorders with onset specific to childhood**
Mainly exaggerations of normal developmental trends rather than phenomena
that are qualitatively abnormal in themselves. Developmental appropriateness is
used as the key diagnostic feature in defining the difference between these emotional disorders, with onset specific to childhood, and the neurotic disorders
(F40–F48).

*Excludes:* • when associated with conduct disorder (F92.–)

*F93.0  Separation anxiety disorder of childhood*
Should be diagnosed when fear of separation constitutes the focus of the anxiety

and when such anxiety first arose during the early years of childhood. It is differentiated from normal separation anxiety when it is of a degree (severity) that is statistically unusual (including an abnormal persistence beyond the usual age period), and when it is associated with significant problems in social functioning.

*Excludes:*  • mood [affective] disorders (F30–F39)
              • neurotic disorders (F40–F48)
              • phobic anxiety disorder of childhood (F93.l)
              • social anxiety disorder of childhood (F93.2)

### F93.1  Phobic anxiety disorder of childhood
Fears in childhood that show a marked developmental phase specificity and arise (to some extent) in a majority of children, but that are abnormal in degree. Other fears that arise in childhood but that are not a normal part of psychosocial development (for example agoraphobia) should be coded under the appropriate category in section F40–F48.

*Excludes:*  • generalized anxiety disorder (F41.1)

### F93.2  Social anxiety disorder of childhood
In this disorder there is a wariness of strangers and social apprehension or anxiety when encountering new, strange, or socially threatening situations. This category should be used only where such fears arise during the early years, and are both unusual in degree and accompanied by problems in social functioning.

Avoidant disorder of childhood or adolescence

### F93.3  Sibling rivalry disorder
Some degree of emotional disturbance usually following the birth of an immediately younger sibling is shown by a majority of young children. A sibling rivalry disorder should be diagnosed only if the degree or persistence of the disturbance is both statistically unusual and associated with abnormalities of social interaction.

Sibling jealousy

### F93.8  Other childhood emotional disorders
Identity disorder
Overanxious disorder
*Excludes:*  • gender identity disorder of childhood (F64.2)

### F93.9  Childhood emotional disorder, unspecified

### F94  Disorders of social functioning with onset specific to childhood and adolescence
A somewhat heterogeneous group of disorders that have in common abnormalities in social functioning which begin during the developmental period, but

which (unlike the pervasive developmental disorders) are not primarily characterized by an apparently constitutional social incapacity or deficit that pervades
all areas of functioning. In many instances, serious environmental distortions or
privations probably play a crucial role in etiology.

### F94.0 Elective mutism

Characterized by a marked, emotionally determined selectivity in speaking, such
that the child demonstrates a language competence in some situations but fails to
speak in other (definable) situations. The disorder is usually associated with
marked personality features involving social anxiety, withdrawal, sensitivity, or
resistance.

Selective mutism

*Excludes:* • pervasive developmental disorders (F84.–)
 • schizophrenia (F20.–)
 • specific developmental disorders of speech and language (F80.–)
 • transient mutism as part of separation anxiety in young children
 (F93.0)

### F94.1 Reactive attachment disorder of childhood

Starts in the first five years of life and is characterized by persistent abnormalities in the child's pattern of social relationships that are associated with emotional disturbance and are reactive to changes in environmental circumstances (e.g.
fearfulness and hypervigilance, poor social interaction with peers, aggression
towards self and others, misery, and growth failure in some cases). The syndrome probably occurs as a direct result of severe parental neglect, abuse, or
serious mishandling.

   Use additional code, if desired, to identify any associated failure to thrive or
growth retardation.

*Excludes:* • Asperger's syndrome (F84.5)
 • disinhibited attachment disorder of childhood (F94.2)
 • maltreatment syndromes (T74.–)
 • normal variation in pattern of selective attachment
 • sexual or physical abuse in childhood, resulting in psychosocial
 problems (Z61.4–Z61.6)

### F94.2 Disinhibited attachment disorder of childhood

A particular pattern of abnormal social functioning that arises during the first
five years of life and that tends to persist despite marked changes in environmental circumstances, e.g. diffuse, nonselectively focused attachment behaviour,
attention-seeking and indiscriminately friendly behaviour, poorly modulated
peer interactions; depending on circumstances there may also be associated
emotional or behavioural disturbance.

Affectionless psychopathy

Institutional syndrome

*Excludes:* • Asperger's syndrome (F84.5)
• hospitalism in children (F43.2)
• hyperkinetic disorders (F90.–)
• reactive attachment disorder of childhood (F94.l)

### F94.8 Other childhood disorders of social functioning

### F94.9 Childhood disorder of social functioning, unspecified

## F95    Tic disorders

Syndromes in which the predominant manifestation is some form of tic. A tic is an involuntary, rapid, recurrent, nonrhythmic motor movement (usually involving circumscribed muscle groups) or vocal production that is of sudden onset and that serves no apparent purpose. Tics tend to be experienced as irresistible but usually they can be suppressed for varying periods of time, are exacerbated by stress, and disappear during sleep. Common simple motor tics include only eye-blinking, neck-jerking, shoulder-shrugging, and facial grimacing. Common simple vocal tics include throat-clearing, barking, sniffing, and hissing. Common complex tics include hitting oneself, jumping, and hopping. Common complex vocal tics include the repetition of particular words, and sometimes the use of socially unacceptable (often obscene) words (coprolalia), and the repetition of one's own sounds or words (palilalia).

### F95.0 Transient tic disorder

Meets the general criteria for a tic disorder but the tics do not persist longer than 12 months. The tics usually take the form of eye-blinking, facial grimacing, or head-jerking.

### F95.1 Chronic motor or vocal tic disorder

Meets the general criteria for a tic disorder, in which there are motor or vocal tics (but not both), that may be either single or multiple (but usually multiple), and last for more than a year.

### F95.2 Combined vocal and multiple motor tic disorder [de la Tourette]

A form of tic disorder in which there are, or have been, multiple motor tics and one or more vocal tics, although these need not have occurred concurrently. The disorder usually worsens during adolescence and tends to persist into adult life. The vocal tics are often multiple with explosive repetitive vocalizations, throat-clearing, and grunting, and there may be the use of obscene words or phrases. Sometimes there is associated gestural echopraxia which may also be of an obscene nature (copropraxia).

*F95.8  Other tic disorders*

*F95.9  Tic disorder, unspecified*
Tic NOS

F98     ***Other behavioural and emotional disorders with onset usually occurring in
childhood and adolescence***
A heterogeneous group of disorders that share the characteristic of an onset in
childhood but otherwise differ in many respects. Some of the conditions represent well-defined syndromes but others are no more than symptom complexes
that need inclusion because of their frequency and association with psychosocial
problems, and because they cannot be incorporated into other syndromes.

> *Excludes:*  • breath-holding spells (R06.8)
> • gender identity disorder of childhood (F64.2)
> • Kleine-Levin syndrome (G47.8)
> • obsessive-compulsive disorder (F42.–)
> • sleep disorders due to emotional causes (F51.–)

*F98.0  Nonorganic enuresis*
A disorder characterized by involuntary voiding of urine, by day and by night,
which is abnormal in relation to the individual's mental age, and which is not a
consequence of a lack of bladder control due to any neurological disorder, to
epileptic attacks, or to any structural abnormality of the urinary tract. The enuresis may have been present from birth or it may have arisen following a period of
acquired bladder control. The enuresis may or may not be associated with a more
widespread emotional or behavioural disorder.

Enuresis (primary)(secondary) of nonorganic origin
Functional enuresis
Psychogenic enuresis
Urinary incontinence of nonorganic origin
*Excludes:*  • enuresis NOS (R32)

*F98.1  Nonorganic encopresis*
Repeated, voluntary or involuntary passage of faeces, usually of normal or near-
normal consistency, in places not appropriate for that purpose in the individual's
own sociocultural setting. The condition may represent an abnormal continuation of normal infantile incontinence, it may involve a loss of continence following the acquisition of bowel control, or it may involve the deliberate deposition
of faeces in inappropriate places in spite of normal physiological bowel control.
The condition may occur as a monosymptomatic disorder, or it may form part of
a wider disorder, especially an emotional disorder (F93.–) or a conduct disorder
(F91.–).

Functional encopresis

Incontinence of faeces of nonorganic origin

Psychogenic encopresis

Use additional code, if desired, to identify the cause of any coexisting constipation.

*Excludes:* • encopresis NOS (R15)

### F98.2 *Feeding disorder of infancy and childhood*

A feeding disorder of varying manifestations usually specific to infancy and early childhood. It generally involves food refusal and extreme faddiness in the presence of an adequate food supply, a reasonably competent caregiver, and the absence of organic disease. There may or may not be associated rumination (repeated regurgitation without nausea or gastrointestinal illness).

Rumination disorder of infancy

*Excludes:* • anorexia nervosa and other eating disorders (F50.–)

           feeding:

           • difficulties and mismanagement (R63.3)

           • problems of newborn (P92.–)

           pica of infancy or childhood (F98.3)

### F98.3 *Pica of infancy and childhood*

Persistent eating of non-nutritive substances (such as soil, paint chippings, etc.). It may occur as one of many symptoms that are part of a more widespread psychiatric disorder (such as autism), or as a relatively isolated psychopathological behaviour; only the latter is classified here. The phenomenon is most common in mentally retarded children and, if mental retardation is also present, F70–F79 should be selected as the main diagnosis.

### F98.4 *Stereotyped movement disorders*

Voluntary, repetitive, stereotyped, nonfunctional (and often rhythmic) movements that do not form part of any recognized psychiatric or neurological condition. When such movements occur as symptoms of some other disorder, only the overall disorder should be recorded. The movements that are of a non self-injurious variety include: body-rocking, head-rocking, hair-plucking, hair-twisting, finger-flicking mannerisms, and hand-flapping. Stereotyped self-injurious behaviour includes repetitive head-banging, face-slapping, eye-poking, and biting of hands, lips or other body parts. All the stereotyped movement disorders occur most frequently in association with mental retardation (when this is the case, both should be recorded). If eye-poking occurs in a child with visual impairment, both should be coded: eye-poking under this category and the visual condition under the appropriate somatic disorder code.

Stereotype/habit disorder

*Excludes:* • abnormal involuntary movements (R25.–)

- movement disorders of organic origin (G20–G25)
- nail-biting (F98.8)
- nose-picking (F98.8)
- stereotypies that are part of a broader psychiatric condition (F00–F95)
- thumb-sucking (F98.8)
- tic disorders (F95.–)
- trichotillomania (F63.3)

### F98.5 Stuttering [stammering]

Speech that is characterized by frequent repetition or prolongation of sounds or syllables or words, or by frequent hesitations or pauses that disrupt the rhythmic flow of speech. It should be classified as a disorder only if its severity is such as to markedly disturb the fluency of speech.

*Excludes:* • cluttering (F98.6)
  • tic disorders (F95.–)

### F98.6 Cluttering

A rapid rate of speech with breakdown in fluency, but no repetitions or hesitations, of a severity to give rise to diminished speech intelligibility. Speech is erratic and dysrhythmic, with rapid jerky spurts that usually involve faulty phrasing patterns.

*Excludes:* • stuttering (F98.5)
  • tic disorders (F95.–)

### F98.8 Other specified behavioural and emotional disorders with onset usually occurring in childhood and adolescence

Attention deficit disorder without hyperactivity
Excessive masturbation
Nail-biting
Nose-picking
Thumb-sucking

### F98.9 Unspecified behavioural and emotional disorders with onset usually occurring in childhood and adolescence

## Unspecified mental disorder (F99)

### F99 Mental disorder, not otherwise specified

Mental illness NOS

*Excludes:* • organic mental disorder NOS (F06.9)

**Other conditions from ICD-10 often associated with mental and behavioural disorders (selected A00–E90 and G00–Y98 categories)**

This section contains a list of conditions in other chapters of ICD-10 that are often found in association with the disorders in Chapter V(F) itself. The majority of the conditions covered are given only at the three-character level, but four-character codes are given for a selection of those diagnoses that will be used most frequently.

*Chapter I*    *Certain infectious and parasitic diseases (A00–B99)*

*A50  Congenital syphilis*

*A50.4  Late congenital neurosyphilis [juvenile neurosyphilis]*

*A52  Late syphilis*

*A52.1  Symptomatic neurosyphilis*
*Includes*:   • tabes dorsalis

*A81  Slow virus infections of central nervous system*

*A81.0  Creutzfeldt-Jakob disease*

*A81.1  Subacute sclerosing panencephalitis*

*A81.2  Progressive multifocal leukoencephalopathy*

*B22  Human immunodeficiency virus (HIV) disease resulting in other specified diseases*

*B22.0  HIV disease resulting in encephalopathy*
*Includes*:   • HIV dementia

*Chapter II*    *Neoplasms (C00–D48)*

*C70.–  Malignant neoplasm of meninges*

*C71.–  Malignant neoplasm of brain*

*C72.–  Malignant neoplasm of spinal cord, cranial nerves and other parts of central nervous system*

*D33.–  Benign neoplasm of brain and other parts of central nervous system*

*D42.– Neoplasm of uncertain and unknown behaviour of meninges*

*D43.– Neoplasm of uncertain and unknown behaviour of brain and central nervous system*

**Chapter IV**     *Endocrine, nutritional and metabolic diseases (E00–E90)*

*E00.– Congenital iodine-deficiency syndrome*

*E01.– Iodine-deficiency-related thyroid disorders and allied conditions*

*E02 Subclinical iodine-deficiency hypothyroidism*

*E03 Other hypothyroidism*

*E03.2 Hypothyroidism due to medicaments and other exogenous substances*

*E03.5 Myxoedema coma*

*E05.– Thyrotoxicosis [hyperthyroidism]*

*E15 Nondiabetic hypoglycaemic coma*

*E22 Hyperfunction of pituitary gland*

*E22.0 Acromegaly and pituitary gigantism*

*E22.1 Hyperprolactinaemia*
*Includes*: • drug-induced hyperprolactinaemia

*E23.– Hypofunction and other disorders of pituitary gland*

*E24.– Cushing's syndrome*

*E30 Disorders of puberty, not elsewhere classified*

*E30.0 Delayed puberty*

*E30.1 Precocious puberty*

*E34 Other endocrine disorders*

*E34.3 Short stature, not elsewhere classified*

*E51  Thiamine deficiency*

*E51.2  Wernicke's encephalopathy*

*E64.–  Sequelae of malnutrition and other nutritional deficiencies*

*E66.–  Obesity*

*E70  Disorders of aromatic amino-acid metabolism*

*E70.0  Classical phenylketonuria*

*E71  Disorders of branched-chain amino-acid metabolism and fatty-acid metabolism*

*E71.0  Maple-syrup-urine disease*

*E74.–  Other disorders of carbohydrate metabolism*

*E80.–  Disorders of porphyrin and bilirubin metabolism*

*Chapter VI*    *Diseases of the nervous system (G00–G99)*

*G00.–  Bacterial meningitis, not elsewhere classified*
*Includes*:   • haemophilus, pneumococcal, streptococcal, staphylococcal and
              other bacterial meningitis

*G02.–  Meningitis in other infectious and parasitic diseases classified elsewhere*

*G03.–  Meningitis due to other and unspecified causes*

*G04.–  Encephalitis, myelitis and encephalomyelitis*

*G06  Intracranial and intraspinal abscess and granuloma*

*G06.2  Extradural and subdural abscess, unspecified*

*G10  Huntington's disease*

*G11.–  Hereditary ataxia*

*G20  Parkinson's disease*

*G21  Secondary parkinsonism*

*G21.0  Malignant neuroleptic syndrome*

*G21.1  Other drug-induced secondary parkinsonism*

*G21.2  Secondary parkinsonism due to other external agents*

*G21.3  Postencephalitic parkinsonism*

**G24  Dystonia**
*Includes*:  • dyskinesia

*G24.0  Drug-induced dystonia*

*G24.3  Spasmodic torticollis*

*G24.8  Other dystonia*
*Includes*:  • tardive dyskinesia

**G25.–  Other extrapyramidal and movement disorders**
*Includes*:  • restless legs syndrome, drug-induced tremor, myoclonus, chorea, tics

**G30  Alzheimer's disease**

*G30.0  Alzheimer's disease with early onset*

*G30.1  Alzheimer's disease with late onset*

*G30.8  Other Alzheimer's disease*

*G30.9  Alzheimer's disease, unspecified*

**G31  Other degenerative diseases of nervous system, not elsewhere classified**

*G31.0  Circumscribed brain atrophy*
*Includes*:  • Pick's disease

*G31.1  Senile degeneration of brain, not elsewhere classified*

*G31.2  Degeneration of nervous system due to alcohol*
*Includes*: • alcoholic cerebellar ataxia and degeneration, cerebral degeneration and encephalopathy; dysfunction of the autonomic nervous system due to alcohol

*G31.8  Other specified degenerative diseases of the nervous system*
*Includes*:  • Subacute necrotizing encephalopathy [Leigh] grey-matter degeneration [Alpers]

*G31.9  Degenerative disease of nervous system, unspecified*

**G32.– Other degenerative disorders of nervous system in diseases classified elsewhere**

**G35  Multiple sclerosis**

**G37  Other demyelinating diseases of central nervous system**

*G37.0  Diffuse sclerosis*
*Includes*:    • periaxial encephalitis; Schilder's disease

**G40  Epilepsy**

*G40.0  Localization-related (focal) (partial) idiopathic epilepsy and epileptic*
    *syndromes with seizures of localized onset*
*Includes*:    • benign childhood epilepsy with centrotemporal EEG spikes or
    occipital EEG paroxysms

*G40.1  Localization-related (focal) (partial) symptomatic epilepsy and epileptic*
    *syndromes with simple partial seizures*
*Includes*:    • attacks without alteration of consciousness

*G40.2  Localization-related (focal) (partial) symptomatic epilepsy and epileptic*
    *syndromes with complex partial seizures*
*Includes*:    • attacks with alteration of consciousness, often with automatisms

*G40.3  Generalized idiopathic epilepsy and epileptic syndromes*

*G40.4  Other generalized epilepsy and epileptic syndromes*
*Includes*:    • salaam attacks

*G40.5  Special epileptic syndromes*
*Includes*:    • epileptic seizures related to alcohol, drugs and sleep deprivation

*G40.6  Grand mal seizures, unspecified (with or without petit mal)*

*G40.7  Petit mal, unspecified, without grand mal seizures*

**G41.– Status epilepticus**

**G43.– Migraine**

**G44.– Other headache syndromes**

**G45.– Transient cerebral ischaemic attacks and related syndromes**

**G47  Sleep disorders**

*G47.2  Disorders of the sleep-wake schedule*

*G47.3  Sleep apnoea*

*G47.4  Narcolepsy and cataplexy*

**G70  Myasthenia gravis and other myoneural disorders**

*G70.0  Myasthenia gravis*

**G91.– Hydrocephalus**

**G92  Toxic encephalopathy**

**G93  Other disorders of brain**

*G93.1  Anoxic brain damage, not elsewhere classified*

*G93.3  Postviral fatigue syndrome*
*Includes:* • benign myalgic encephomyelitis

*G93.4  Encephalopathy, unspecified*

**G97  Postprocedural disorders of nervous system, not elsewhere classified**

*G97.0  Cerebrospinal fluid leak from spinal puncture*

**Chapter VII**  **Diseases of the eye and adnexa (H00–H59)**

**H40  Glaucoma**

*H40.6  Glaucoma secondary to drugs*

**Chapter VIII**  **Diseases of the ear and mastoid process (H60–H95)**

**H93  Other disorders of ear, not elsewhere classified**

*H93.1  Tinnitus*

*Chapter IX*     *Diseases of the circulatory system (I00–I99)*

*I10  Essential (primary) hypertension*

*I60.–  Subarachnoid haemorrhage*

*I61.–  Intracerebral haemorrhage*

*I62  Other nontraumatic intracranial haemorrhage*

*I62.0  Subdural haemorrhage (acute) (nontraumatic)*

*I62.1  Nontraumatic extradural haemorrhage*

*I63.–  Cerebral infarction*

*I64  Stroke, not specified as haemorrhage or infarction*

*I65.–  Occlusion and stenosis of precerebral arteries, not resulting in cerebral infarction*

*I66.–  Occlusion and stenosis of cerebral arteries, not resulting in cerebral infarction*

*I67  Other cerebrovascular diseases*

*I67.2  Cerebral atherosclerosis*

*I67.3  Progressive vascular leukoencephalopathy*
*Includes*:   • Binswanger's disease

*I67.4  Hypertensive encephalopathy*

*I69.–  Sequelae of cerebrovascular disease*

*I95  Hypotension*

*I95.2  Hypotension due to drugs*

*Chapter X*     *Diseases of the respiratory system (J00–J99)*

*J10  Influenza due to identified influenza virus*

*J10.8  Influenza with other manifestations, influenza virus identified*

*J11  Influenza, virus not identified*

*J11.8  Influenza with other manifestations, virus not identified*

*J42  Unspecified chronic bronchitis*

*J43.–  Emphysema*

*J45.–  Asthma*

*Chapter XI*     *Diseases of the digestive system (K00–K93)*

*K25  Gastric ulcer*

*K26  Duodenal ulcer*

*K27  Peptic ulcer, site unspecified*

*K29  Gastritis and duodenitis*

*K29.2  Alcoholic gastritis*

*K30  Dyspepsia*

*K58.–  Irritable bowel syndrome*

*K59.–  Other functional intestinal disorders*

*K70.–  Alcoholic liver disease*

*K71.–  Toxic liver disease*
*Includes*:   • drug-induced liver disease

*K86  Other diseases of pancreas*

*K86.0  Alcohol-induced chronic pancreatitis*

*Chapter XII*     *Diseases of the skin and subcutaneous tissue (L00–L99)*

*L20.–  Atopic dermatitis*

*L98  Other disorders of skin and subcutaneous tissue, not elsewhere classified*

*L98.1  Factitial dermatitis*
*Includes*:   • neurotic excoriation

*Chapter XIII*     **Diseases of the musculoskeletal system and connective tissue (M00–M99)**

**M32.– Systemic lupus erythematosus**

**M54.– Dorsalgia**

*Chapter XIV*     **Diseases of the genitourinary system (N00–N99)**

**N48  Other disorders of penis**

**N48.3  Priapism**

*N48.4  Impotence of organic origin*

**N91.– Absent, scanty and rare menstruation**

**N94  Pain and other conditions associated with female genital organs and menstrual cycle**

*N94.3  Premenstrual tension syndrome*

*N94.4  Primary dysmenorrhoea*

*N94.5  Secondary dysmenorrhoea*

*N94.6  Dysmenorrhoea, unspecified*

**N95  Menopausal and other perimenopausal disorders**

*N95.1  Menopausal and female climacteric states*

*N95.3  States associated with artificial menopause*

*Chapter XV*     **Pregnancy, childbirth and the puerperium (O00–O99)**

**O04  Medical abortion**

**O35  Maternal care for known or suspected fetal abnormality and damage**

*O35.4  Maternal care for (suspected) damage to fetus from alcohol*

*O35.5  Maternal care for (suspected) damage to fetus by drugs*

**O99  Other maternal diseases classifiable elsewhere but complicating pregnancy, childbirth and puerperium**

*O99.3  Mental disorders and diseases of the nervous system complicating pregnancy, childbirth and the puerperium*

*Includes*:   • conditions in F00–F99 and G00–G99

***Chapter XVII***   ***Congenital malformations, deformations, and chromosomal abnormalities (Q00–Q99)***

**Q02  Microcephaly**

**Q03.–  Congenital hydrocephalus**

**Q04.–  Other congenital malformations of brain**

**Q05.–  Spina bifida**

**Q75.–  Other congenital malformations of skull and face bones**

**Q85  Phakomatoses, not elsewhere classified**

*Q85.0  Neurofibromatosis (nonmalignant)*

*Q85.1  Tuberous sclerosis*

**Q86  Congenital malformation syndromes due to known exogenous causes, not elsewhere classified**

*Q86.0  Fetal alcohol syndrome (dysmorphic)*

**Q90  Down's syndrome**

*Q90.0  Trisomy 21, meiotic nondisjunction*

*Q90.1  Trisomy 21, mosaicism (mitotic nondisjunction)*

*Q90.2  Trisomy 21, translocation*

*Q90.9  Down's syndrome, unspecified*

*Q91.– Edwards' syndrome and Patau's syndrome*

*Q93  Monosomies and deletions from the autosomes, not elsewhere classified*

*Q93.4  Deletion of short arm of chromosome 5*
*Includes*:   • cri-du-chat syndrome

*Q96.– Turner's syndrome*

*Q97.– Other sex chromosome abnormalities, female phenotype, not elsewhere*
*classified*

*Q98  Other sex chromosome abnormalities, male phenotype, not elsewhere classified*

*Q98.0  Klinefelter's syndrome karyotype 47, XXY*

*Q98.1  Klinefelter's syndrome, male with more than two X chromosomes*

*Q98.2  Klinefelter's syndrome, male with 46, XX karyotype*

*Q98.4  Klinefelter's syndrome, unspecified*

*Q99.– Other chromosome abnormalities, not elsewhere classified*

*Chapter XVIII  Symptoms, signs and abnormal clinical and laboratory findings, not elsewhere*
*classified (R00–R99)*

*R55  Syncope and collapse*

*R56  Convulsions, not elsewhere classified*

*R56.0  Febrile convulsions*

*R56.8  Other and unspecified convulsions*

*R62  Lack of expected normal physiological development*

*R62.0  Delayed milestone*

*R62.8  Other lack of expected normal physiological development*

*R62.9  Lack of expected normal physiological development, unspecified*

*R63  Symptoms and signs concerning food and fluid intake*

*R63.0  Anorexia*

*R63.1  Polydipsia*

*R63.4  Abnormal weight loss*

*R63.5  Abnormal weight gain*

**R78.–  Findings of drugs and other substances, normally not found in blood**
*Includes:*  • alcohol (R78.0); opiate drug (R78.1); cocaine (R78.2); hallucinogen (R78.3); other drugs of addictive potential (R78.4); psychotropic drug (R78.5); abnormal level of lithium (R78.8)

**R83  Abnormal findings in cerebrospinal fluid**

**R90.–  Abnormal findings on diagnostic imaging of central nervous system**

**R94  Abnormal results of function studies**

*R94.0  Abnormal results of function studies of central nervous system*
*Includes:*  • abnormal electroencephalogram [EEG]

*Chapter XIX*  **Injury, poisoning and certain other consequences of external causes (S00–T98)**

**S06  Intracranial injury**

*S06.0  Concussion*

*S06.1  Traumatic cerebral oedema*

*S06.2  Diffuse brain injury*

*S06.3  Focal brain injury*

*S06.4  Epidural haemorrhage*

*S06.5  Traumatic subdural haemorrhage*

*S06.6  Traumatic subarachnoid haemorrhage*

*S06.7  Intracranial injury with prolonged coma*

*Chapter XX*   **External causes of morbidity and mortality (V0I–Y98)**

**Intentional self-harm (X60–X84)**
*Includes*: • purposely self-inflicted poisoning or injury; suicide

**X60  Intentional self-poisoning by and exposure to nonopioid analgesics, antipyretics and antirheumatics**

**X61  Intentional self-poisoning by and exposure to antiepileptic, sedative-hypnotic, antiparkinsonism and psychotropic drugs, not elsewhere classified**
*Includes*:  antidepressants, barbiturates, neuroleptics, psychostimulants

**X62  Intentional self-poisoning by and exposure to narcotics and psychodysleptics [hallucinogens], not elsewhere classified**
*Includes*: • cannabis (derivatives), cocaine, codeine, heroin, lysergide [LSD], mescaline, methadone, morphine, opium (alkaloids)

**X63  Intentional self-poisoning by and exposure to other drugs acting on the autonomic nervous systems**

**X64  Intentional self-poisoning by and exposure to other and unspecified drugs and biological substances**

**X65  Intentional self-poisoning by and exposure to alcohol**

**X66  Intentional self-poisoning by and exposure to organic solvents and halogenated hydrocarbons and their vapours**

**X67  Intentional self-poisoning by and exposure to other gases and vapours**
*Includes*: • carbon monoxide; utility gas

**X68  Intentional self-poisoning by and exposure to pesticides**

**X69  Intentional self-poisoning by and exposure to other and unspecified chemicals and noxious substances**
*Includes*: • corrosive aromatics, acids and caustic alkalis

**X70  Intentional self-harm by hanging, strangulation and suffocation**

**X71  Intentional self-harm by drowning and submersion**

**X72  Intentional self-harm by handgun discharge**

**X73  Intentional self-harm by rifle, shotgun and larger firearm discharge**

*X74  Intentional self-harm by other and unspecified firearm discharge*

*X75  Intentional self-harm by explosive material*

*X76  Intentional self-harm by fire and flames*

*X77  Intentional self-harm by steam, hot vapours and hot objects*

*X78  Intentional self-harm by sharp object*

*X79  Intentional self-harm by blunt object*

*X80  Intentional self-harm by jumping from a high place*

*X81  Intentional self-harm by jumping or lying before moving object*

*X82  Intentional self-harm by crashing of motor vehicle*

*X83  Intentional self-harm by other specified means*
*Includes*: • crashing of aircraft, electrocution, caustic substances (except poisoning)

*X84  Intentional self-harm by unspecified means*

*Assault (X85–Y09)*
*Includes*: • homicide; injuries inflicted by another person with intent to injure or kill, by any means

*X93  Assault by handgun discharge*

*X99  Assault by sharp object*

*Y00  Assault by blunt object*

*Y04  Assault by bodily force*

*Y05  Sexual assault by bodily force*

*Y06.–  Neglect and abandonment*

*Y07.–  Other maltreatment syndromes*
*Includes*: • mental cruelty; physical abuse; sexual abuse; torture

*Drugs, medicaments and biological substances causing adverse effects in therapeutic use (Y40–Y59)*

*Y46  Antiepileptics and antiparkinsonism drugs*

*Y46.7 Antiparkinsonism drugs*

*Y47.– Sedatives, hypnotics and antianxiety drugs*

*Y49  Psychotropic drugs, not elsewhere classified*

*Y49.0  Tricyclic and tetracyclic antidepressants*

*Y49.1  Monoamine-oxidase-inhibitor antidepressants*

*Y49.2  Other and unspecified antidepressants*

*Y49.3  Phenothiazine antipsychotics and neuroleptics*

*Y49.4  Butyrophenone and thioxanthene neuroleptics*

*Y49.5  Other antipsychotics and neuroleptics*

*Y49.6  Psychodysleptics [hallucinogens]*

*Y49.7  Psychostimulants with abuse potential*

*Y49.8  Other psychotropic drugs, not elsewhere classified*

*Y49.9  Psychotropic drug, unspecified*

*Y50.– Central nervous system stimulants, not elsewhere classified*

*Y51.– Drugs primarily affecting the autonomic nervous system*

*Y57.– Other and unspecified drugs and medicaments*

# Two

# Axis Two  WHO Short Disability Assessment Schedule (WHO DAS-S)

1.     *PERIOD COVERED BY RATING*    (tick appropriate box):

   ☐    current

   ☐    last month

   ☐    last year

   ☐    other (specify): _____

2.     *SPECIFIC AREAS OF FUNCTIONING*    (circle appropriate figure):

   **A.**    *Personal care*

   Refers to personal hygiene, dressing, feeding, etc.

   (no disability)     0    1    2    3    4    5    (gross disability)

   ☐    functioning with assistance

   **B.**    *Occupation*

   Refers to functioning in paid activities, studying, homemaking, etc.

   (no disability)     0    1    2    3    4    5    (gross disability)

   ☐    functioning with assistance

**C.     Family and household**

Refers to interaction with spouse, parents, children and other relatives, participation in household activities, etc. In rating, pay particular attention to performance in the context in which the individual lives.

(no disability)      0    1    2    3    4    5      (gross disability)

☐     functioning with assistance

**D.     Functioning in broader social context**

Refers to expected performance in relation to community members, participation in leisure and other social activities.

(no disability)      0    1    2    3    4    5      (gross disability)

☐     functioning with assistance

3.      *TOTAL DURATION OF DISABILITY* (tick appropriate box):

☐     less than 1 year
☐     1 year or more
☐     unknown

4.      *SPECIFIC ABILITIES*

Some patients may get a high rating of disability in one or more of the above areas, but may nevertheless have specific abilities that are important for the management of care and individual's functioning in the community or family. Such an asset may be the skilful handling of a musical instrument, particularly good looks, physical strength or ease in social situations.

Tick if specific abilities are present and describe:

☐     ...........................................................................

...........................................................................

# Axis Three

## Listing and brief definitions of selected ICD-10 Z categories and specific Z codes

**Z61–Z62    Problems related to negative events in childhood and upbringing**

*Z61.0    Loss of love relationship in childhood*
Loss of an emotionally close relationship, such as of a parent, a sibling, a very special friend or a loved pet, by death or permanent departure or rejection.

*Z61.1    Removal from home in childhood*
Prolonged involuntary stay away from home such as in a foster home, hospital or other institution causing psychosocial distress.

*Z61.3    Events resulting in loss of self-esteem in childhood*
Events resulting in a negative self-reappraisal by the child such as failure in tasks with high personal investment; disclosure or discovery of a shameful or stigmatizing personal or family event; and other severely humiliating experiences.

*Z61.6    Problems related to alleged physical abuse of child*
Problems related to incidents in which the child has been injured in the past by any adult in the household to a medically significant extent (e.g., fractures, marked bruising) or that involved excessive forms of violence (e.g., burning or tying up of the child, prolonged starvation, confinement in a small space).

*Z61.7    Personal frightening experience in childhood*
Experience carrying a threat for the child's future, such as a kidnapping, natural disaster with a threat to life, injury with a threat to self-image or security, or witnessing a severe trauma to a loved one.

*Z61.8    Other specified negative life events in childhood*

*Z62.0    Inadequate parental supervision and control*
Lack of parental knowledge of what the child is doing or where the child is; poor control over the child's socially undesirable activities; lack of concern or lack of attempted intervention when the child is in risky or dangerous situations.

Three

### Z62.1    Parental overprotection
Pattern of upbringing that discourages the child's own initiative, independent decision-making and spontaneous behaviour.

### Z62.2    Institutional upbringing
Group foster care in which parenting responsibilities are largely taken over by some form of institution (such as a residential nursery, orphanage, or children's home).

### Z62.4    Emotional neglect of child
Inadequate emotional care of the child for prolonged duration including lack of interest in the child, of sympathy for the child's difficulties and of praise and encouragement, cold and aloof attitude towards the child.

### Z62.5    Other problems related to neglect in upbringing
Lack of opportunities for learning and playing, prolonged uncertainties about availability of food, shelter or clothing.

### Z62.8    Other specified problems related to upbringing

## Z55    Problems related to education and literacy

### Z55.0    Illiteracy or low-level literacy
Complete lack or low level of ability to read and write.

### Z55.1    Schooling unavailable or unattainable
Lack of opportunity to attend school because of its unavailability or other practical difficulties such as distance or cost.

### Z55.2    Failed examinations
Repeated failures in examinations (not directly caused by an Axis I disorder).

### Z55.3    Underachievement in school
Failure to fulfil the educational expectations, taking into consideration the socio-cultural background and the intellectual ability.

### Z55.4    Educational maladjustment and discord with teachers and classmates
Inadequacy in adapting to the educational system and repeated or prolonged interrelational problems with teachers and/or classmates.

### Z55.8    Other specified problems related to education and literacy (e.g. inadequate teaching)

**Z63**   **Problems related to primary support group, including family circumstances**

*Z63.0   Problems in relationship with spouse or partner*
Repeated or prolonged interpersonal problems between the partners resulting in significantly disturbed family atmosphere.

*Z63.1   Problems in relationship with parents or in-laws*
Repeated or prolonged interpersonal problems with parents or in-laws resulting in significantly disturbed family atmosphere.

*Z63.2   Inadequate family support*
Lack of family support to the extent that it causes psychosocial distress to the individual.

*Z63.3   Absence of family member*
Prolonged absence of a family member causing psychosocial distress to the individual.

*Z63.4   Disappearance or death of family member; assumed death of family member*
Death of a family member or his/her prolonged and unexplained disappearance assumed to be caused by death.

*Z63.5   Disruption of family by separation or divorce*
Prolonged or indefinite separation between partners or divorce between the spouses leading to significant disruption of the family and estrangement between partners.

*Z63.6   Dependent relative needing care at home*
A member of the family needing significant help in activities of daily living at home.

*Z60.1   Atypical parenting situation*
Problems related to parenting situation other than of two biological parents living together, e.g. single parent, adoptive parents, same-sex parent.

*Z63.7   Other stressful life events affecting family and household*
Serious physical or mental (including psychoactive substance use) disorders within the family, isolated family.

*Z63.8   Other specified problems related to the primary support group*

**Z60    Problems related to the social environment**

*Z60.2    Living alone*
Living without partner, spouse or any other family member.

*Z60.3    Acculturation difficulty*
Problems related to adaptation and living in a different culture including migration and social transplantation.

*Z60.4    Social exclusion and rejection*
Exclusion and rejection on the basis of personal characteristics, such as unusual physical appearance, illness, behaviour or habits.

*Excludes:*  • target of adverse discrimination such as for racial or religious reasons (Z60.5)

*Z60.5    Target of perceived adverse discrimination and persecution*
Persecution or discrimination, perceived or real, on the basis of membership of some group (as defined by skin colour, religion, ethnic origin, etc.) rather than personal characteristics.

*Excludes:*  • social exclusion and rejection (Z60.4)

*Z60.8    Other specified problems related to social environment*

**Z59    Problems related to housing or economic circumstances**

*Z59.0    Homelessness*
Not having a home to live in, living on the street.

*Z59.1    Inadequate housing or residential institution*
Lack of adequate and essential necessities in the home or residential institution including inadequate space, inadequate protection from the environment (e.g., lack of heating), inadequate privacy or unsatisfactory surroundings.

*Excludes:*  • problems related to physical environment (Z58.-)

*Z59.2    Discord with neighbours, lodgers or landlords*
Repeated or prolonged interpersonal problems with neighbours, lodgers or landlords.

*Z59.3    Problems related to living in residential institution*
Problems related to the living circumstances in the residential institution such as boarding school, hostel, home for the elderly.

*Excludes:*  • institutional upbringing (Z62.2)

*Z59.5   Extreme poverty*
Not having enough money to manage even the bare necessities of life.

*Z59.6   Insufficient income to cover daily needs*
Not having enough money to manage the daily needs satisfactorily.

*Z59.7   Insufficient social insurance and welfare support*
Lack of adequate help from the community to manage satisfactorily.

*Z59.8   Other problems related to housing and economic circumstances*

## Z56   Problems related to (un)employment

*Z56.0   Unemployment*
Lack of gainful employment in spite of willingness to work.

*Z56.1   Change of job*
Change in the nature or place of work or of employer.

*Z56.2   Threat of job loss*
Events or situations which are threatening for the continuation of gainful employment.

*Z56.3   Stressful work schedule*
Problems related to timing or irregularity of work hours.

*Z56.4   Discord with boss and workmates*
Repeated or prolonged interpersonal problems with superiors and/or co-workers.

*Z56.5   Uncongenial work*
Nature of work, working conditions or other charcteristics of work perceived as sufficiently adverse to cause significant problems.

*Z56.6   Other specified physical or mental strain related to work (e.g. discrimination at work place, harassment at work place, dangerous work environment)*

## Z57–Z58   Problems related to physical environment

*Z57   Occupational exposure to risk factors*
Exposure to a physical environment capable of causing harm in the occupational setting, e.g. high levels of noise, radiation, dust, or toxic agents in agriculture or industry.

*Z58    Non-occupational exposure to physical environment*
Exposure to a physical environment capable of causing harm in a non-occupational setting, e.g., high level of noise, radiation, dust, toxic agents, heat or cold.

## Z64    Problems related to certain psychosocial circumstances

*Z64.0    Problems related to unwanted pregnancy*
Psychosocial problems directly arising from a current pregnancy that is perceived by the pregnant woman as unwanted.

*Z64.1    Problems related to multiparity*
Psychosocial problems directly arising from having had numerous childbirths.

*Z64.4    Discord with counsellors, probation officers, social workers, etc.*
Repeated or prolonged interpersonal problems with community services functionaries, social agencies or community service personnel, e.g., counsellors, probation officers, social workers, etc.

## Z65    Problems related to legal circumstances

*Z65.0    Conviction in civil or criminal proceeding without imprisonment*
Conviction by a court of law in a civil or criminal case but not leading to imprisonment.

*Z65.1    Imprisonment or other incarceration*
Imprisonment due to conviction and sentence by a court of law in civil or criminal case. Also includes other sentences involving involuntary stay in an institution under legal orders.

*Z65.3    Problems related to other legal circumstances*
Problems related to involvement with the legal system such as arrest for an alleged crime, civil or criminal legal proceedings, child custody or support care.

*Z65.4    Victim of crime, terrorism or torture*
Circumstances in which the individual involuntarily becomes a victim of criminal activities, terrorism or deliberate torture.

*Z65.5    Exposure to disaster, war or other hostilities*
Circumstances in which the individual gets significantly affected by natural or man-made disasters, war or other incidents involving threat to a large number of individuals.

**Z81-Z82     Problems related to family history of diseases or disabilities**

*Z81     Family history of mental or behavioural disorders*
A positive family history of mental or behavioural disorders including family history of alcohol abuse or dependence; tobacco abuse or dependence; and other psychoactive substance abuse or dependence.

*Z82     Family history of physical disabilities and chronic physical diseases*
A positive family history of physical disabilities and chronic physical diseases suchä as: epilepsy or other diseases of the nervous system; blindness and visual loss; deafness or hearing loss; stroke; ischemic heart disease; other diseases of the circulatory system; asthma or other chronic lower respiratory diseases; arthritis or other diseases of the musculoskeletal system and connective tissue; congenital malformations, deformations or chromosomal abnormalities; or other disabilities and chronic diseases leading to disability not elsewhere classified.

**Z72     Lifestyle and life-management problems (in the absence of a respective Axis I disorder)**

*Z72.0     Tobacco use (excludes tobacco dependence)*
Use of tobacco in a manner that influences the Axis I condition, but is insufficient to fulfill the criteria for an Axis I disorder.

*Z72.1     Alcohol use (excludes alcohol dependence)*
Use of alcohol in a manner that influences the Axis I condition, but is insufficient to fulfill the criteria for an Axis I disorder.

*Z72.2     Drug use (excludes abuse of non-dependence producing substances and drug dependence)*
Use of drugs in a manner that influences the Axis I condition, but is insufficient to fulfill the criteria for an Axis I disorder.

*Z72.3     Lack of physical exercise*
Insufficient or inadequate everyday physical activity or exercise to an extent that is likely to lead to adverse health effects.

*Z72.4     Inappropriate diet or eating habits*
Content of diet or eating habits are inappropriate to an extent that they are likely to lead to adverse health effects.

*Z72.5     High risk sexual behaviour*
Sexual behaviour that is likely to lead to significant health risks to the individual and/or others.

**Z72.8** *Other specified problems related to lifestyle (e.g., irregular or inappropriate sleeping patterns)*

**Z73.0** *Burn-out*
State of emotional exhaustion, disillusionment and withdrawal with reduced feeling of personal accomplishment in certain type of professionals (e.g., various caregivers).

**Z73.1** *Accentuation of personality traits (in the absence of a respective Axis I disorder)*
Accentuation of the individual's characteristic and enduring patterns of inner experience and behaviour, that are not adequate or sufficient for diagnosis of an adult personality disorder, e.g., Type A behaviour pattern (unbridled ambition, a need for high achievement, importance, competitiveness, and a sense of urgency)

**Z73.2** *Lack of relaxation and leisure*
Insufficient or inadequate relaxation and lack of leisure activities not directly caused by an Axis I disorder.

**Z73.3** *Stress, not elsewhere classified*
Any environmental incident that requires change in ongoing life adjustment and produces the stress reaction, i.e., the physiological, behavioural and subjective responses to the incident.

**Z73.4** *Inadequate social skills, not elsewhere classified*
Inability to fulfill the social norms and expectations taking account of the individual's sociocultural context.

**Z73.5** *Social role conflict, not elsewhere classified*
Experience of conflict due to the individual exhibiting behaviour/attitudes that are incompatible with his/her role in a given sociocultural context.

**Z73.8** *Other specified life-management problems*

# Index

Each entry is followed by a roman numeral, which indicates the axis to which that category belongs, and the ICD-10 code for the category.

Page numbers are given in *italics*.

## ICD-10 Multiaxial Diagnostic Formulation Form

Patient's name or ID code: _____ Age (years): _____ Sex (M/F): _____

Clinician's name or ID code: _____ Institution: _____

Date of assessment (D/M/Y): ___/___/___

Assessment time frame (circle one): current/last month/last year/other (specify): _____

### Axis I: Clinical Diagnoses

*List all positive diagnoses and enter respective ICD-10 codes. Record both mental and physical disorders and conditions here. Enter the principal diagnosis first. Use listing of the ICD-10 diagnoses and categories provided in Part II.*

| Diagnoses | ICD-10 A-Y codes |
|---|---|
| 1. | |
| 2. | |
| 3. | |
| 4. | |
| 5. | |

### Axis II: Disabilities

*Rate disabilities from 0-5 in each of the specific areas of functioning using WHO DAS-S, which is provided in Part II. Transfer ratings here.*

| Disabilities in specific areas of functioning | Ratings (0-5) |
|---|---|
| A. Personal care | |
| B. Occupation | |
| C. Family and household | |
| D. Broader social context | |

Functioning with assistance in following areas (circle all appropriate): A B C D
Specific abilities (specify if present): ..........................................

### Axis III: Contextual factors

*List all present contextual factors and enter specific Z codes for each. Include only factors of significant influence on occurrence, presentation, course, outcome or treatment of disorders recorded on Axis I, or factors of clear relevance for clinical care of patient's condition. List contextual factors in order of importance. Use attached listing of contextual factors and ICD-10 Z codes provided in Part II .*

| Contextual factors | ICD-10 Z codes |
|---|---|
| 1. | |
| 2. | |
| 3. | |
| 4. | |
| 5. | |

Printed in the United States
By Bookmasters